Kettlebells
FOR
DUMMIES®

by Sarah Lurie, RKC, CSCS

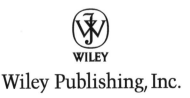

WILEY

Wiley Publishing, Inc.

Kettlebells For Dummies®

Published by
Wiley Publishing, Inc.
111 River St.
Hoboken, NJ 07030-5774
www.wiley.com

For general information on our other products and services, please contact our Customer Care Department within the U.S. at 877-762-2974, outside the U.S. at 317-572-3993, or fax 317-572-4002.

For technical support, please visit www.wiley.com/techsupport.

Wiley also publishes its books in a variety of electronic formats. Some content that appears in print may not be available in electronic books.

Library of Congress Control Number: 2010926848

ISBN: 978-0-470-59929-7

ISBN 978-0-470-59929-7 (pbk); ISBN 978-0-470-76938-6 (ebk); ISBN 978-0-470-76939-3 (ebk); ISBN 978-0-470-76940-9 (ebk)

Manufactured in the United States of America

10 9 8 7 6 5 4 3

WILEY

About the Author

In October 2004, **Sarah Lurie** founded Iron Core, the first kettlebell training studio in the country to exclusively offer Russian Kettlebell Challenge (RKC) certified kettlebell instruction. Lurie is a former fitness competitor and did traditional weight training for more than ten years before discovering kettlebells. After experiencing a debilitating injury during a workout, Lurie discovered that kettlebell training helped her overcome her injury and get back into a comprehensive fitness routine.

Lurie is a nationally recognized kettlebell expert and has been featured in *The New York Times, The Wall Street Journal, Fitness Magazine, Oxygen Magazine, Women's Health, Reader's Digest,* and *Newsweek*. She has appeared on *E! News, The Big Idea* with Donny Deutsch, *Better Homes and Gardens TV, Home Shopping Network* (HSN), and numerous local television fitness programs. Her at-home workout DVDs are sold at retailers nationwide.

Lurie earned a BA in Economics from the University of Arizona and a Masters in Public Administration from San Diego State University. She lives with her husband and two daughters in San Diego.

Dedication

For my husband Jesse, daughters Emma and Grace, and P.A.L. Thanks for teaching me love, patience, persistence, courage, commitment, and dedication (among many other things!). And, of course, Emma, your 3 a.m. wake-up calls made this book possible.

For my dad, who believed in me from the day we drew the logo on the napkin together.

For my mom and Garth for all your encouragement over the years.

Author's Acknowledgments

It all started with the RKC in Minneapolis in June 2004. I will always be grateful to visionaries John DuCane and Pavel Tsatsouline for bringing the training modality and equipment to the United States. Thank you to Brett Jones for being my mentor for the first two-and-a-half (formative) years of my career. Your willingness to share your knowledge and your precise training helped shape my career.

This book would not have been possible without the help of Mark Reichenthal. Thanks for believing in me enough to recommend that I author this book.

The team at Wiley has been an absolute pleasure to work with. Thank you to Tracy Boggier, my acquisitions editor, for all your positive encouragement through the trial writing process. My project editor, Georgette Beatty, is top notch and always provided the support, encouragement, and attention to detail that I needed to get this project done — thank you. Thank you to my copy editor, Amanda Langferman, and my technical reviewer, Andrea U-Shi Chang, for your hard work — your attention to detail was invaluable to this project.

Over the years, I've been lucky enough to work with some incredibly talented and caring RKCs, most of whom began as clients. I want to thank all the Iron Core RKCs for continually being dedicated to your trade and to our clients. Thank you to Osvaldo Aponte, Cody Bramlett, Charlie Fields, Jessie Shea, Farrah Lin, Elizabeth Sansone, and Denise Holsapple — Iron Core would not continue to exist without all of you. I have to give a special thank-you to Osvaldo Aponte. Os is not only one of the most dedicated and talented instructors I've worked with, but he's also my incredibly patient trainer, who helped me stay in shape during both of my pregnancies and got me back into fighting shape after baby Emma. Os, thank you for taking over when I no longer could be there and for keeping the energy of the gym alive.

I could not have gotten through the process of completing this book without the help and expertise of Rochelle Lewis — thank you for your patience and professionalism.

Along the way, too, I have worked with some incredible clients who have always given me encouragement and support throughout the years. Thank you to Carol Raymond (my very first client), Jackie Harris, Cookie Holsapple, Holly Kennedy, Mike Wasser, Lynne-Sharpe Underwood, and all the others from the original Iron Core crew.

Thank you to Osvaldo Aponte, Erica Buechner, Lynne-Sharpe Underwood, Maddy James, and Mike Byergo for your patience and professionalism as models for this book.

Thank you to Davia Matson, my makeup artist for the book, for getting rid of my dark circles.

A special thanks to Maurice Roy, who has been my photographer since I started Iron Core. Your photos make the instructions in the book come alive.

Last but certainly not least, I am grateful to the readers of this book. Thank you for purchasing the book and for wanting to learn how to use kettlebells!

Publisher's Acknowledgments

We're proud of this book; please send us your comments at http://dummies.custhelp.com. For other comments, please contact our Customer Care Department within the U.S. at 877-762-2974, outside the U.S. at 317-572-3993, or fax 317-572-4002.

Some of the people who helped bring this book to market include the following:

Acquisitions, Editorial, and Media Development

Senior Project Editor: Georgette Beatty

Acquisitions Editor: Tracy Boggier

Copy Editor: Amanda M. Langferman

Assistant Editor: Erin Calligan Mooney

Senior Editorial Assistant: David Lutton

Technical Editor:
Andrea U-Shi Chang, RKC, CK-FMS

Editorial Manager: Michelle Hacker

Editorial Assistant: Jennette ElNaggar

Art Coordinator: Alicia B. South

Cover Photo: Sarah Lurie

Cartoons: Rich Tennant
(www.the5thwave.com)

Composition Services

Project Coordinator: Katherine Crocker

Layout and Graphics: Brent Savage, Joyce Haughey, Christine Williams

Special Art: Photos © Maurice Roy Photography; Illustrations by Kathryn Born, M.A.

Proofreaders: Lindsay Littrell, Linda Seifert

Indexer: Rebecca Salerno

Publishing and Editorial for Consumer Dummies

Kathleen Nebenhaus, Vice President and Executive Publisher

Kristin Ferguson-Wagstaffe, Product Development Director

Ensley Eikenburg, Associate Publisher, Travel

Kelly Regan, Editorial Director, Travel

Publishing for Technology Dummies

Andy Cummings, Vice President and Publisher

Composition Services

Debbie Stailey, Director of Composition Services

Contents at a Glance

Table of Contents

Table of Contents   *xiii*

The two-kettlebell windmill...171
Correcting your windmill form with a partner exercise..............173
The One-Arm Row..174
The Renegade Row with One Kettlebell..................................176
The High Pull...177
The Single-Leg Dead Lift..180
Doing the single-leg dead lift with two hands on the kettlebell......180
Trying a one-handed variation of the single-leg dead lift............182
Performing a corrective exercise for the single-leg dead lift........182
The Tactical Lunge..184
The Deck Squat..186
Performing the basic deck squat......................................186
Using different methods to help you perform
   the deck squat successfully..187

Chapter 11: Whittle Your Middle: Core Exercises 189

The Hot Potato..190
The Seated Russian Twist..192
The Renegade Row with Two Kettlebells.................................193
Putting It All Together: A 15-Minute Core Circuit.....................195

Chapter 12: Mastering the Five Ultimate Kettlebell Exercises 197

The Clean and Jerk..198
The Snatch..200
The Overhead Squat..203
The basic overhead squat...203
Corrective drills for the overhead squat.............................204
The Sots Press..206
The Pistol: The Ultimate in Leg and Glute Strength...................207
The pistol without a kettlebell......................................207
The pistol with a kettlebell...208
Fixing form with the assisted pistol.................................210
Building Endurance and Strength with Five
Fiery Five-Minute Workouts..211
Workout 1: Leg- and glute-endurance builder..........................211
Workout 2: Upper-body strengthener and
   cardio-endurance builder...212
Workout 3: Upper- and lower-body strengthener........................212
Workout 4: Lower-body strengthener and
   cardio-endurance builder...213
Workout 5: Cardio-endurance builder and fat burner...................213

**Chapter 13: Kicking It Up a Notch with Advanced
Kettlebell Workouts and Combinations. 215**

Advanced Workout 1: Flab to Fab......................................216
Advanced Workout 2: Cardio Burn......................................218
Advanced Workout 3: Power and Strength...............................220

Introduction

The biggest question on your mind when you picked up this book may have been, "What exactly are kettlebells?" Simply stated, kettlebells are weights that look like cannonballs with handles; exercising with them combines strength training and cardio training into one workout. Using kettlebells has been hailed in recent years as the most efficient and effective way to train your body for burning tons of fat, getting super strong and lean, and obtaining the ultimate physique. Professional athletes, Hollywood stars, fitness enthusiasts, and novice exercisers have all found in kettlebells what they couldn't find in other workouts — an exercise program that can be done in half the time of a regular workout routine with twice the results.

I got involved with kettlebells when they were still in their infancy — not many people had heard of Russian kettlebells back in 2003, and very few qualified kettlebell instructors, books, or workout DVDs existed. However, since that time, kettlebell training has grown by leaps and bounds; major fitness organizations recognize it not only as a legitimate training tool but also as one of the best tools available for getting lean and strong. Many qualified trainers now teach students across the country how to use kettlebells. And university research studies are beginning to surface, proving what Russian kettlebell expert Pavel Tsatsouline and his first wave of kettlebell enthusiasts knew all along — kettlebells are the ultimate exercise tool for anyone who's willing to put in the time to learn how to use them and isn't afraid of a little sweat.

About This Book

My goal in this book is to use both photos and step-by-step instruction to explain precisely and concisely how to use kettlebells, beginning with the most fundamental principles (such as proper form for your spine and hips). I guide you through a number of basic exercises to help you start using your kettlebell properly, quickly, and safely, and I help you progress to more advanced moves to help you get the absolute most out of your exercise time.

In addition, although I wrote this book with the novice in mind, those of you who have used kettlebells before can find plenty of useful information that you may have missed when you first started using kettlebells — nuances on form and technique that can make a big difference in the results you get from your routine. I also include information on advanced moves to take your workout to the next level and pointers for special audiences who want to use kettlebells, such as young adults, baby boomers, seniors, pregnant women, and others.

And keep in mind that you don't have to read this book from cover to cover; I've organized this book so you can dip into and out of it to find the information you need when you need it.

Conventions Used in This Book

The instructions in this book are meant to be simple, yet comprehensive, to help you establish proper form and technique from the very beginning of your kettlebell practice. With that in mind, I use the following conventions to help you navigate through the information easily:

- ✔ For most of the fundamental kettlebell exercises, I walk you through the basics of the exercise without using your kettlebell before I explain how to do it using your kettlebell.

- ✔ I include at least two photos (and in some cases three or more) with the majority of the exercises in this book so you can see what each stage of the exercise looks like.

- ✔ I include opportunities for you to practice your technique and form after I explain how to do each exercise by providing you with a practice set of reps.

- ✔ I write all instructions and explanations in nontechnical terms so that you aren't bogged down by unfamiliar language; whenever necessary, I use *italics* to point out new terms or add emphasis.

- ✔ I present step-by-step instructions in **boldface** to help you easily identify what you need to know to properly execute the exercise.

 Any extra explanatory text that helps you get a better handle on a particular step appears in roman text after the boldface step.

- ✔ I use monofont to make Web sites stand out.

 When this book was printed, some Web addresses may have needed to break across two lines of text. If that happened, rest assured that I haven't put in any extra characters (such as hyphens) to indicate the break. So, when using one of these Web addresses, just type in exactly what you see in this book, pretending as though the line break doesn't exist.

What You're Not to Read

This book is packed full of detailed information that explains how to use kettlebells, and it's based on my experience of teaching new students how to use kettlebells for the first time. I certainly won't object if you read this book from cover to cover, but if necessary, you can safely skip anything marked with an Advanced Stuff icon; you can also skip sidebars (in shaded gray boxes). These items contain interesting information but aren't crucial to understanding how to use kettlebells.

Foolish Assumptions

As I wrote this book, I made a few assumptions about you. Basically, I assumed the following:

✔ You're a novice when it comes to kettlebells. In other words, you've either heard of or read about kettlebells and may have watched clips of other people using them, but either have never touched a kettlebell or recently bought one and don't know what to do with it.

✔ If you have used kettlebells and are self-taught, you may be lacking in some areas of your form and technique. For you, the instructions I present in this book will provide clarification on what you already know — and will undoubtedly make a big difference in the results you get from your kettlebell routine.

✔ You possess little fitness experience and are looking for a workout routine that's fun and challenging and that gets results; oh, and you aren't afraid of elevating your heart rate and working your muscles!

How This Book Is Organized

Kettlebells For Dummies is organized into five parts with each part offering you detailed information on specific topics related to kettlebells. The following sections explain what each part covers.

Part 1: Gearing Up for a Kettlebell Workout

Part I gives you an overview of kettlebell training and explains how it differs from traditional fitness programs. It provides information on the benefits of kettlebell training, the reasons why it works, and essential safety considerations you need to take before and during your workouts. Knowing what size kettlebell to start with and how to pick the right quality kettlebell is a subject that many newbies have trouble with, so I dedicate an entire chapter to helping you pick the right kettlebell and set up a safe and effective home gym. In addition, Part I details essential hip, spine, and breathing techniques to get you moving and using your kettlebell properly, and it offers warm-up and cool-down options to help you start and finish your workouts safely.

Part II: Beginning with Basic Kettlebell Moves

Part II is one of the most important parts of the book because it shows you how to build the foundation for your entire kettlebell practice. It's full of step-by-step instructions that take you through the fundamental kettlebell exercises, like the swing and the Turkish get-up. For each exercise, you find valuable information on how to fix your form or technique if you're having trouble with the exercise. You also find some basic workout routines that allow you to start practicing right away with a cohesive workout program (after you master the basics, of course!).

Part III: Mastering Advanced Kettlebell Moves

When you're ready to kick your kettlebell workouts up a notch, take a look at Part III; it offers intermediate and advanced moves to help you keep your workout challenging. In addition, it covers some great abdominal-specific exercises that work your core even more than the advanced full-body kettlebell exercises do. Be forewarned, though, this part contains five ultimate kettlebell exercises that will take your training to a whole new level — with a little time and patience, of course! To help you put the exercises I cover in this part together into an effective (and challenging) workout routine, I offer a few workout options for you to try out at the end of this part.

Part IV: Using Kettlebells in Special Situations

Over the years, I've been lucky enough to work with a variety of individuals at different life stages and fitness levels. Whether you're a young adult, a baby boomer or senior, a pregnant woman, an athlete, or someone who's overweight or rehabbing from an injury, you find what you need to know in this part to adapt your kettlebell workout to your particular situation. Kettlebells are a highly adaptable tool if they're used correctly. In this part, I use a conservative approach to help you incorporate a few kettlebell exercises into your specific workout routine, but, as you gain confidence with kettlebells, you'll find that the rest of this book is just as helpful as this particular part.

Part V: The Part of Tens

A signature of *For Dummies* books, the Part of Tens contains lists of ten things you may want to know about kettlebells. Chapter 18 details ten ways you can set and meet your kettlebell fitness goals, and Chapter 19 points out ten tips for working with a kettlebell trainer. The appendix lists resources to help you find anything and everything you may need related to kettlebells, including a list of certified trainers near you.

Icons Used in This Book

The icons in this book are true to *For Dummies* style and point out especially useful tidbits of information. Here's a list of the icons I use in this book:

This icon points out important information that you should take away from this book and apply to every kettlebell workout you do.

This icon points out nuances and variations on form and technique that can help make the exercises easier.

This icon alerts you to some essential information on safe form and technique. Read the information attached to this icon so you don't hurt yourself!

If you master a basic exercise and feel ready to progress, use the information highlighted with this icon to guide you in doing more challenging variations.

Where to Go from Here

If you're a beginner and just want to dive right in, flip to Chapter 2 to take note of some important safety considerations you need to follow, Chapter 3 to choose the right size kettlebell, and Chapter 4 to begin with some spine and hip essentials. Then be sure to read Chapter 5 on warming up, cooling down, and breathing right before attempting the basic exercises in Chapters 6, 7, and 8.

If you've used kettlebells before, you may still want to take a look at Chapters 4 and 5 to make sure you're using the right form and techniques in your exercises. Then feel free to move on to Parts II and III, where you can start working on basic and, eventually, more advanced kettlebell exercises.

If you fall into any of the special-situation categories in Part IV, begin with Chapters 4 and 5, and then skip to the appropriate chapter on your particular situation, where you can find the guidance you need to get started.

No matter where you fall on the fitness spectrum, kettlebells will help you achieve your fitness, health, and wellness goals. As you start your kettlebell fitness journey, get ready to be encouraged with some instant results: your skin will feel firmer, your posture will improve, and you'll have more energy for life's everyday challenges. After you commit to a workout schedule, within weeks, you'll notice more positive changes. For example, you'll feel stronger, your clothes will begin to fit better, you'll have more endurance, and your friends and family will probably ask you what you've been doing differently. I've seen some remarkable results from my clients who have committed themselves to learning and practicing kettlebells. Use this book to begin your journey to achieving your ultimate body — and don't forget, I'll be with you every step of the way!

Part I
Gearing Up for a Kettlebell Workout

The 5th Wave   By Rich Tennant

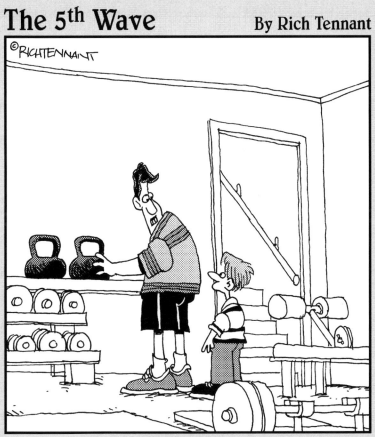

"A kettlebell? Imagine something the weight of a bowling ball only with a handle, like Mommy's purse."

In this part . . .

1f you're ready to get moving with kettlebells, you're in the right place. In this part, you find information on what kettlebells are, the benefits your body gets from a kettlebell workout, and the important safety considerations you need to keep in mind as you train. If you want to find out what size kettlebell to use, get the scoop on where to buy it, and determine how many bells you need, look no further — this part has all these answers, too.

To be successful with a kettlebell workout program, you need to know how to align your spine and move your hips as well as how to warm up, cool down, and breathe properly. Lucky for you, this part is here to show you how to do all this and more.

Chapter 1

Shaping Up with Kettlebells

Welcome to the world of kettlebells! A kettlebell, which looks like a cannonball with a handle, is a very simple, yet effective piece of equipment that allows you to work most of your muscle groups at the same time. Because of the fast-paced, dynamic motions in kettlebell exercises, your heart rate increases with each repetition, keeping your body in the fat-burning zone throughout your workout.

One of the greatest things about using kettlebells is that you don't need to be a hard-core, experienced fitness enthusiast to start using them. However, if you want to get the results that a kettlebell offers, you do have to challenge and tax your muscles and cardiovascular strength. Kettlebells are a tough, no-nonsense workout tool that will challenge you both physically and mentally. So, if you're someone who prefers to read your paper on the treadmill, kettlebells are probably not a good choice for you. On the other hand, if you're someone who enjoys being challenged when you work out, you'll surely find success with kettlebells. As you become a more experienced kettlebeller, you'll be pushed to your limit as you swing and snatch your way to a stronger and more confident you.

In this chapter, I introduce you to some kettlebell fundamentals, including how kettlebells are different from other workouts and how to move your spine and hips properly when using them. I also describe a sampling of basic exercises, show you where to go if you're ready to advance to more challenging exercises, and note how special audiences can work out with kettlebells. Prepare to get moving!

Comparing Kettlebells to Other Workouts

Kettlebell exercise is different from traditional weight lifting and other fitness programs in many ways. For example,

- ✓ **Kettlebells combine a strength-training and cardiovascular workout into one program.** Very few workout programs accomplish such a combination, and those that do aren't accessible to or easily learned by the novice. Olympic lifting comes close to the power and strength you get from working out with kettlebells, but it lacks the versatility of kettlebells. Ever try swinging a barbell between your legs? Besides, Olympic lifts aren't nearly as easy to learn as kettlebell exercises. And I don't know about you, but I don't have any desire to squat 400 pounds on a regular basis.

- ✓ **Most kettlebell exercises utilize all your major muscle groups.** A kettlebell workout doesn't isolate muscle groups, so instead of working just one muscle group like you do with a dumbbell, kettlebells work multiple muscle groups with each exercise. The result is a workout that's quicker, more efficient, and more effective than a traditional workout routine.

Check out Chapter 2 to find out more about the benefits of working out with kettlebells and how to use them safely.

Selecting Your Kettlebell and Gathering Other Gear

One very appealing aspect of kettlebell workouts is that you don't need much equipment to do them. One kettlebell is all you need to start with, and, if you choose the correct size at the beginning, you won't have to go and buy another one for a while. Plus, even when you are ready to move up in kettlebell weight, you'll still have uses for your lighter kettlebell (such as during warm-up exercises that involve the kettlebell; see Chapter 5). Typically, experienced kettlebellers (or those who just want to try a few of the two-kettlebell workouts like the ones I provide in this book) have two or three kettlebells, but even so, relative to some other fitness programs, kettlebells are an inexpensive fitness tool. Refer to Chapter 3 for a complete discussion on how to pick the right size kettlebell and where to get one.

The only other gear besides your kettlebell that you really need to get started is a stopwatch, a yoga mat (or some sort of padded flooring like carpet), and this book. Any other equipment listed throughout the book is optional, and I give you plenty of alternatives for using items you probably already have in your house (like a chair) so you can get started right away. And it's okay if you haven't purchased your kettlebell just yet, because, with most of the foundational exercises, I help you practice without your kettlebell before I show you how to do the exercise with your kettlebell.

Getting a Grip on Proper Spine and Hip Alignment

When it comes to using kettlebells the right way, you need to take some time to figure out how to position your spine and move from your hips to maximize the benefit you get from your workout and minimize the chance of injury. The majority of people I've trained over the years don't know how to position their spine and hips properly when they take their first kettlebell class because most traditional exercises don't incorporate these essential principles. Here's one big example: People who perform squat exercises in the gym typically use a machine to assist them, and, when they squat, their range of motion is limited.

However, when you squat down to the floor to pick up a box or some other object (like a kettlebell), not only do you need a greater range of motion than a typical squat requires of your body, but you also need to know how to initiate the movement from your hips (so you don't hurt your back), how to brace your abdominals (so you stabilize your core for strength and control throughout the movement), and how to press through your heels to activate your glutes and hamstrings (see Chapter 4 for more details). Kettlebells help you master these basic techniques and show you that moving in this way is actually very natural.

I can't emphasize enough how the essential techniques in Chapter 4 will benefit your body and get you moving for success. There, you find the details on achieving *neutral spine* (the natural *S* curve in your back) and snapping your hips the right way so you're properly aligned throughout all your kettlebell workouts.

Breathing Correctly, Warming Up, Cooling Down, and Easing Up

Mastering the right breathing technique is an essential part of using kettlebells properly. But, don't worry — it isn't as technical as it sounds. In fact, breathing the right way for kettlebells comes quite naturally, and after you know how to use the right breathing pattern during your exercises, your breathing in everyday life will feel much more powerful and less shallow.

The technique I recommend is called *diaphragmatic breathing,* and it's simply a way to tighten your *virtual belt* — which is also known as abdominal bracing. Using this breathing technique allows you to protect yourself from the weight and force of your kettlebell before you even execute an exercise by stabilizing your core with breath control.

In addition, like any fitness program, warming up, cooling down, and making sure you haven't overdone it are important parts of being successful with your routine.

- ✔ You can use dynamic stretches and Z-Health options during your warm-up; you can also incorporate your kettlebell into your warm-up.

- ✔ To cool down, you can do some quick 'n' easy stretches as well as use a band and a foam roller.

- ✔ If you find yourself sore after a workout, you can try some simple techniques to ease the soreness; if you've really gone overboard, you need to modify your program for success.

Make sure to read through Chapter 5 to figure out how to breathe, warm up, and cool down properly and how to relieve muscle soreness. (As a bonus in that chapter, I also discuss some options for making your workout's rest periods a little more active.)

Starting with Basic Exercises

To begin your kettlebell practice, you need to learn a few basic foundational exercises. If you take the time to hone these basic movements, you'll find it much easier to learn more intermediate and advanced exercises, not to mention you'll be less likely to develop bad habits in form and technique. Starting with the basic exercises I cover in Chapters 6 through 8 (and introduce in the following sections) is necessary for you to get above-average results from your kettlebell workout — and speaking of workouts, I provide a few full-length routines built from these basics in Chapter 9.

The swing

The swing is the first foundational exercise I walk you through in this book, and it has many variations. However, you need to master only three basic variations to have a well-rounded kettlebell routine:

✔ **Two-arm swing:** The most basic swing exercise, this variation requires you to have two hands on the kettlebell when moving it.

✔ **One-arm swing:** As you probably guessed, this variation involves moving the kettlebell with only one hand on it.

✔ **Alternating swing:** For this slightly more advanced variation, you have to switch your hand positioning while the kettlebell is "live" or in the air.

None of these variations is particularly difficult to execute; in fact, the basic movement in the swing is quite natural. Its benefits include trimming and strengthening your core and rear, building cardiovascular endurance, and burning lots of fat. Refer to Chapter 6 for complete details on performing swings.

The Turkish get-up

Although the Turkish get-up is considered a basic exercise, it's one of the most difficult exercises to master. The good news is that you can break down the Turkish get-up into manageable steps, so you can master one part of the movement at a time and then put them together as you go. Before you know it, you'll be performing the complete exercise flawlessly.

Even though doing this exercise well takes some practice, like the swing, it's an important foundational exercise to master. The Turkish get-up shows you how to keep your shoulders sunk into their sockets, which is an essential principle in all kettlebell exercises. The Turkish get-up also has many other benefits — developing shoulder and core stability and increasing shoulder mobility, just to name a couple. Chapter 7 offers a comprehensive lesson on how to master the Turkish get-up and its variations.

The front squat, the clean, and the military press

The front squat, the clean, and the military press round out the foundational exercises. After you master the swing, doing the squat, the clean, and the press is somewhat simpler because you already know how to move the kettlebell with your hips, maintain proper spine alignment, and follow other important principles that carry over to these exercises. The squat, the clean, and the press all strengthen your core, help slim your waist and glutes, increase your mobility and flexibility, and build cardiovascular and muscular endurance. See Chapter 8 for the fundamentals of these three moves.

Moving to Advanced Exercises

To make progress with your kettlebell workout, you have to continue to challenge your body. Sometimes my workouts consist of only the five basic exercises that I describe in the preceding section, but most workouts have at least one or two intermediate-to-advanced exercises in them, too. Here's where to go to get more info:

- ✔ Check out Chapter 10 to find exercises that take your training beyond the basics with moves specifically meant to improve your strength, flexibility, and mobility.
- ✔ Turn to Chapter 11 for some abdominal-specific exercises that focus on working your core even more than the other kettlebell moves.
- ✔ Go to Chapter 12 for details on how to do the five ultimate kettlebell exercises that test your body from head to toe and further increase your strength and cardiovascular endurance.

To wrap up, Chapter 13 provides a few routines built from these advanced exercises (with a few basic exercises and combinations thrown in for good measure).

Kettlebells for Special Audiences

I address several categories of special audiences in Part IV of this book, and I offer a few variations for exercises so that, no matter what your circumstances are, you can get started right away with your kettlebell routine. These audiences include young adults, baby boomers, and seniors; pregnant women as well as women who have just given birth; athletes of all levels; and people who are rehabbing from injury or in the process of major weight loss.

Young adults, boomers, and seniors

Whether you're a young adult, a baby boomer, or a senior, you can find success with a kettlebell workout. I've worked with all these age groups, and I haven't found much difference between what you can do with kettlebells compared with what someone who's considered an average exerciser can do. Typically, if you fall into one of these categories, the only differences are that you use a lighter weight than the average person and your workouts don't last as long. Some exercises I don't recommend for a beginner young adult, boomer, or senior, but, as time goes on and you get more confident with the workout, most of the exercises in this book will be a good fit for you.

Flip to Chapter 14 for the full scoop on adjusting your kettlebell workout if you're a young adult, a boomer, or a senior.

Pregnant women and women who have just delivered

As I wrote this book, I was pregnant with my second child. I exercised with kettlebells throughout my first pregnancy, used them to melt away the baby fat after my baby was born, and continued to use them during my second pregnancy. Not only have I always felt energetic, strong, and mobile, but I've never experienced any back pain typical of most pregnant women. In addition, I've had lots of strength, energy, and flexibility to keep up with my toddler.

Being pregnant is a wonderful time to begin a workout routine if you haven't already been doing one. As long as your doctor gives you the okay to do strength training during your pregnancy, you'll find so many benefits from exercising regularly; plus, you'll be in the routine of exercising when the baby comes, so you won't have to work as hard to jump right back in post baby. Refer to Chapter 15 for complete guidelines and exercises for when you're either pregnant or looking to get your pre-baby body back after you have the baby.

Athletes of all levels

Athletes of all levels find that kettlebells deliver an incredible endurance- and power-building workout in a very short period of time. If you're a busy athlete, you don't have a lot of time to do fitness programs other than your sport; you need a program that directly carries over and mimics the movements you do in your sport. Because kettlebells build so much core strength, a kettlebell workout transfers completely and immediately to any sport, from track to football and everything in between.

Check out Chapter 16 for pointers on using kettlebells if you're a high-level athlete, a recreational athlete, or just a weekend warrior.

Folks recovering from an injury or undergoing substantial weight loss

If you've gone through rehab and are ready to engage in strength training, kettlebells can be a good alternative to the limiting exercises in traditional weight training. One of the most appealing advantages of using kettlebells to complete your rehabilitation program is that the exercises use full ranges of motion and mimic everyday movements. However, you must have your doctor's okay to use kettlebells to rehab and be conservative in your approach for doing so. Use the guidelines in Chapter 17 to get started.

Here's another scenario to consider: If you have a lot of weight to lose and have tried everything else with no success or just plain hate to exercise, kettlebells may be just what you need. Although using kettlebells effectively will take work and perseverance, you don't find many reasonable and safe exercise programs that burn as many calories in as short amount of time as kettlebells. Plus, kettlebells are easy to use (with the right instructions — which is where I come in), are adaptable to all fitness levels, and, best of all, can be done from the privacy of your own home. Start with the exercises in Chapter 17 and then progress to use the programs throughout the book to continue your weight-loss journey.

Chapter 2

A Primer on Kettlebells: What They Are and How You Use Them

*I*n 2003, when I discovered kettlebells, not many mainstream fitness enthusiasts were using them. Indeed, most people looked at me with a blank stare when I told them I was opening a kettlebell gym. Since then, kettlebell training has become wildly popular among professional athletes, Hollywood stars, and regular folks.

So what exactly are kettlebells and what's their allure? I admit, those big, black cast-iron balls look downright scary! Seriously, though, kettlebells are one of the most powerful and effective training tools to get you strong and fit without requiring you to spend all your free time in the gym. And after you get over how intimidating they look and start swinging one around, you'll probably want to find out more about how to use kettlebells safely and effectively.

An added bonus to kettlebells is that anyone (regardless of age or fitness level) can use them. Over the years, I've helped all types of people at all different fitness levels — from young athletes to senior citizens — master the art of using kettlebells. So, even though the bells themselves may look a bit odd, figuring out how to use them is easy and will make you into a lean, mean, fighting machine in no time. In this chapter, I get you acquainted with kettlebells and their benefits, and I describe a few safety considerations to keep in mind as you begin your training.

Getting to Know Kettlebells

You may not have heard of kettlebells until recently, but they date all the way back to the 1800s when the Russians first used them for exercise. Referred to as handle bells or *girya* in Russia, kettlebells had two main uses: to increase aerobic efficiency and to build strength, power, and endurance. And because they were so effective in these uses, kettlebells found their place in the United States, too. Old-time U.S. strongmen like Arthur Saxon and Eugen Sandow used kettlebells to build very lean, strong bodies — which you can clearly see by looking at any old photos of them!

In the following sections, I describe kettlebells and their differences from other types of weights, and I explain who can use them.

Taking a closer look at what kettlebells are and how they differ from other weights

A kettlebell looks like a cannonball or bowling ball (without the finger holes) with a suitcase handle on the top. A kettlebell's handle and center of gravity are much different from those of a dumbbell or barbell; its design makes it easy to move dynamically and safely around your body. In other words, thanks to the kettlebell's design, your body has to work constantly during both the acceleration and deceleration of any given movement to control and stabilize the weight, and you have to use most of your major muscle groups, especially your core muscles, to do so. Basically, the weight of the kettlebell makes it a strength-training tool, and the fact that you have to constantly control the kettlebell's shifting center of gravity makes kettlebell training one of the toughest and most challenging cardiovascular and core-strengthening workouts around.

You may be wondering why you can't just swing around a dumbbell and call it a day. Here are just a few reasons why doing so isn't a good idea:

✔ The handle of a dumbbell doesn't allow you to move the dumbbell smoothly and rotationally in your hand without the risk of dropping it.

✔ A dumbbell's center of gravity is completely different from a kettlebell's, so you don't get the same core-strengthening or cardiovascular workout.

✔ The awkwardness of trying to use a dumbbell for kettlebell exercises doesn't make for a smooth workout. (Try swinging a 20-kilogram dumbbell between your legs; it isn't easy!)

I understand if you're skeptical — I was too the first time I tried kettlebells. But trust me: They're deceptively effective. You could run on the treadmill for an hour and then lift weights for an hour and still not get the same benefits of a half-hour kettlebell workout. (I describe the various benefits of kettlebell training in detail later in the section "Body Beauty and Strength: Surveying the Benefits of Kettlebell Training.")

Mixing it up: Using kettlebells with other weights

Some people use kettlebells as a stand-alone training tool (one is all you need), but others like to mix some kettlebell exercises into their traditional weight-lifting routines. Why is this combination a good idea? Performing traditional barbell lifts like dead lifts and squats can be great compliments to your kettlebell training. I wasn't originally sold on the idea of kettlebells, but when I mixed three basic kettlebell exercises into my traditional weight-lifting routine, I immediately noticed such a difference in my physique that I soon converted solely to kettlebells.

Identifying who can use kettlebells

Whether you're an athlete, a couch potato, a fitness enthusiast, a grandparent, or someone in between, you fit the profile of people who use kettlebells. Oh, and law enforcement officials, the military, professional athletes, and Hollywood stars also use kettlebells. I myself used kettlebells long before I became a mother and then used them after giving birth to get my pre-baby body back; I continue to use them as I progress through my second pregnancy. You really don't find many people who can't use them. As long as you have a willingness to learn proper form and technique, kettlebells can be a very effective training tool for you.

Kettlebells are a rigorous cardiovascular and strength workout. To ensure your safety, get your doctor's clearance before beginning a kettlebell workout program. (I discuss additional safety considerations in the later section "Keeping a Few Important Safety Considerations in Mind.")

Body Beauty and Strength: Surveying the Benefits of Kettlebell Training

Believe it or not, the first time I did a basic kettlebell exercise (the swing, which I cover in Chapter 6) I thought to myself, "I'm not so sure about this." At the time, I was lifting traditional weights and competing in fitness competitions. But even though I doubted them, kettlebells had a mystique that intrigued me. As I continued to use them, my body changed drastically — I got leaner and stronger, especially in my waist, hips, and rear end (thanks to the combination of cardio and strength training that kettlebells offer).

Kettlebell workouts offer numerous other benefits, too, including the following:

✔ They burn up to 20 calories a minute, and they build your cardiovascular endurance to a high level.

✔ They increase your mobility and flexibility and give you functional strength — strength for real-life movements and situations.

✔ They work all your major muscle groups in a single workout.

✔ They're a multipurpose and versatile fitness tool.

✔ They help you get lean and strong muscles in half the time of a traditional workout — and with less equipment, too!

✔ They challenge you mentally because they involve trying to tame and conquer a piece of iron!

I discuss all these benefits in more detail in the following sections.

Building strength and cardio endurance

Typically, when you go to the gym, you have to do some sort of cardio workout before or after your weight-training routine. Traditional weight-lifting exercises with machines and free weights just don't get your heart rate up to the same level that, say, running on a treadmill does. But doing this type of dual routine can suck up a lot of time and doesn't always produce the desired results.

Perhaps one of the biggest selling points of a kettlebell workout is that it combines a cardio workout and a strength-training workout into one. Because you move the kettlebell so dynamically around your body, your heart rate elevates to a higher level than it would if you were simply isolating body parts with free weights or machines. Performing a dynamic kettlebell exercise for 30 seconds is equivalent to running or sprinting for 30 seconds. This cardio blast, in combination with the fact that you're slinging around a weighted piece of cast iron, makes for one very effective and heart-pounding workout.

Using kettlebells, you get a better and more effective workout in about 30 minutes than you would using traditional weights and isolating muscle groups for an hour — but you must use the right size kettlebell. Flip to Chapter 3 for guidelines on selecting the right size for you.

Working more than just a few of your muscles

Another great benefit of the kettlebell workout is that each exercise taxes a major portion of the body's musculature. In other words, *all* your major muscle groups get a workout with just a single kettlebell exercise.

Consider the foundational exercise, the swing, as an example. When you perform the swing (which I describe in Chapter 6), you work your thighs, hamstrings, glutes, core, and arms — talk about getting the most bang for your buck! Working your muscles in this way trains your muscles to work together as a unit, which greatly increases your body's *functional strength* (in other words, strength for normal life activities). Kettlebells are one of the best ways to train your body to handle life's everyday challenges, such as moving furniture or boxes, carrying groceries or your child, and bending down to pick up something off the floor.

Because you work all your muscles evenly with a kettlebell workout, you can grow incredibly strong without being bulky. Kettlebells have a particularly special allure for women who want to look lean and fit without risking getting big guy-like muscles. I don't know about you, but I like having the confidence that I can carry heavy things without getting help from or resembling a man!

Maintaining interest and increasing strength with its versatility

The kettlebell truly is a multipurpose piece of equipment that yields surprising results. It offers a lot more versatility than a single dumbbell for a variety of reasons. First of all, as I discuss earlier in this chapter, the ability to be able to pass the kettlebell from hand to hand easily and move it dynamically around your body means you can use a kettlebell in many more ways than a dumbbell or a barbell. Secondly, you aren't limited by the weight of your kettlebell (like you are with a dumbbell) because you can continually mix up the repetitions, sets, time, and exercises you do. For example,

- ✔ If you've chosen to use a 26-pound (12-kilogram) kettlebell and it begins to feel too light for the clean and press exercise (see Chapter 8), you can perform a *bottoms-up* version of the exercise (turning the kettlebell upside down so the flat part is facing up toward the ceiling) with the same size kettlebell to create a whole new challenge. In other words, by putting a new twist on an old exercise, you make the same size kettlebell feel like the next size up in weight.

- ✔ If your 26-pound kettlebell begins to feel too light when you perform ten repetitions of the two-arm swing exercise that I describe in Chapter 6, try doing the exercise for one minute. You may be surprised to find that you get an entirely new type of workout with the same size weight.

Using less equipment to do more

Because of the versatility of the kettlebell, you don't need a lot of equipment to see and feel the many effects of your kettlebell routine. Indeed, one kettlebell is all you need for a complete home gym! You can do more with one kettlebell than you can do with a room full of multiple-size free weights. As time goes on, many kettlebell enthusiasts add some additional kettlebells to their collection, but even if you end up with two or three kettlebells, you'll still have less equipment than you would if you wanted to have a complete gym of free weights and a cardio machine. Buying one, two, or three kettlebells costs you a lot less than purchasing all that other stuff, so you have plenty of money left over to buy some really nice workout clothes!

Challenging your mind

Another important benefit of working out with kettlebells is that it continually challenges your mind; each repetition requires that you're completely focused on how you're moving and using your body. Your ability to concentrate and focus on where you feel the movement and how you move with the kettlebell is one of the keys to mastering the exercises. Because you need to be focused on what you're feeling and where you're feeling it (so you don't get hurt), you feel compelled to get better at your form as you practice (which, as you probably guessed, is a whole other challenge!). And you certainly can't ignore the challenge of trying to control and tame a big hunk of iron that moves so dynamically around your body.

Keeping a Few Important Safety Considerations in Mind

The kettlebell workout is a very high-energy, dynamic one, and, like any other workout, you need to master the basics of technique and form properly in order to perform the exercises safely and effectively. In addition, you need to be aware of a few other safety considerations before you start your kettlebell workout routine. Lucky for you, this section is here to tell you all about them and more so that you can get the most out of your kettlebell training program — without getting hurt.

Choosing high-energy workout times and getting plenty of rest between workouts

In general, no time of day is better than any other for working out; however, choosing the time of day when you have the most energy has a big impact on how you perform when working out. On the other hand, if you're tired when you work out, you increase your chances of losing focus and perhaps injuring yourself. For example: If you aren't a morning person, an early morning workout probably isn't the best choice for you. Choose the days and times that work best for you and your body; just be sure to stick with a consistent schedule so you get the best results from your workout routine.

In terms of how long your kettlebell workouts should be, beginners can start with 20- to 30-minute workouts. As you get more proficient and build muscle and cardio endurance, you can add more time to lengthen your workouts, but, in general, a 45-minute kettlebell workout is more than enough time to work all your major muscle groups and tax your cardiovascular system.

How you split the days of your workouts largely depends on your personal schedule. Unlike a traditional weight-lifting routine, you don't necessarily have to split your days according to what body parts you're working. Because the majority of kettlebell exercises work your major muscle groups, a basic three-day-a-week kettlebell program may have you working out on Monday, Wednesday, and Friday or on Tuesday, Thursday, and Saturday. This type of workout routine gives you plenty of time to rest in between workouts. Rest is important because it allows your body to safely execute dynamic kettlebell exercises that require a lot of energy and stamina.

Perhaps you're also a runner or do some other kind of sport or cardio workout and you want to combine your other workouts with your kettlebell routine. In that case, either you can do your other workouts on the days you don't do your kettlebell routine, or you can work out after your kettlebell routine. If you combine kettlebells with another workout routine, listen to your body to make sure you aren't overdoing it. A good rule of thumb is to take off at least one day per week from any exercise when you're combining kettlebells with another workout program.

If you're using the right size kettlebell, you're going to need all the energy you can get for your kettlebell workout (see Chapter 3 for more on how to pick the right size kettlebell). So if you do another type of workout on the same days as your kettlebell routine, perform the kettlebell portion first.

Flip to Chapter 9 for some sample weekly programs; Part IV gives you the scoop on safe workout lengths and frequencies for special audiences (such as young adults, baby boomers, seniors, pregnant women, and others).

Understanding space and flooring requirements

You don't need a ton of space for your kettlebell workouts. A 5-x-5-foot area typically offers plenty of space in which to perform the traditional kettlebell exercises. Keep in mind, though, that if you want to add any body weight exercises (exercises using only your body weight for resistance) or plyometric exercises (fast, explosive movements that usually involve jumping) into your routine, you may want to have a bit more space. No matter the size of your workout area, you need to make sure it's free from clutter, children, pets, or anything else that could distract you or get in your way during your workout.

The flooring surface you choose to use is also an important component of your workout. The ideal flooring surface has just the right amount of firmness and cushion. To achieve this perfect balance, you can put a yoga mat (or similar matting surface) on top of your wood or concrete floor. A yoga mat provides enough cushion for exercises like the Turkish get-up (see Chapter 7) but is also firm enough to allow you to ground yourself properly for exercises like the swing (see Chapter 6). Firm martial-arts mats work well, too.

Knowing what to wear for maximum comfort and movement

The workout clothes and footwear you choose to wear during your kettlebell workouts have a definite impact on how you perform during those workouts. I explain what you need to know in the following sections.

Clothing

A general rule of thumb to follow when you're picking out workout clothes is to choose clothes that allow you to move freely. Here are some guidelines:

- ✔ **Tops:** Wear tops that your body can breath in, like the ones made of fabric designed to move sweat from your skin to the shirt's surface, where it evaporates. Style isn't as important as comfort, so choose the style that makes you feel the most confident and comfortable.

- ✔ **Bottoms:** Short shorts aren't necessary, but baggy ones aren't a good choice, either. Owning a gym in California, I see many male clients who like to wear surfer shorts to class. Baggy shorts or pants impede your performance because they don't allow you to sit back into your hips properly for the majority of kettlebell exercises. So, to get the most out of your workout, be sure to choose a pair of shorts or pants that fits you a little more snugly.

Shoes

Like your workout clothes, the footwear (or lack of it) that you choose to wear during your workouts also affects your performance with kettlebells. I prefer to be barefoot, as do many of my students. Going barefoot or wearing flat-soled shoes, like Vibram FiveFingers or Nike Free shoes, allows your brain to receive feedback from the ground. This contact with the ground is important because you need to be rooted and grounded during all your kettlebell movements. In other words, you need to feel the ground so that your brain knows how to move and use your body for maximum power and efficiency.

If you're wary of going barefoot during your workouts and want to wear shoes, just make sure the shoes you choose are flat-soled sneakers without any sort of elevated heel; a running shoe isn't a good choice. A boxing shoe or one worn during a Pilates class is typically a good option. If you need orthotics or have some other foot condition that requires you to wear a shoe that's different from what I recommend, by all means do so.

Wristbands and other stuff for your hands

Many of my beginning students wear wristbands for added comfort when they're getting used to having the weight of the kettlebell rest on their wrists during exercises like the clean, which involves bringing the bell into the rack position (see Chapter 8). In addition, some students who need to work on technique and form inevitably bang their wrists the first few times when learning exercises like the snatch (see Chapter 12), so wristbands can help alleviate the pressure of the kettlebell.

If you decide to try out a wristband, make sure to buy one that's three inches thick (or thicker); a smaller size doesn't cover enough area on your wrist to be of much help.

When you first begin to do kettlebell exercises, your hands can become calloused, so many of my students have asked me whether they can wear gloves while using the bells. I advise against doing so for a couple of reasons. First of all, wearing gloves actually makes holding onto the kettlebell handle a lot more difficult because the glove makes the grip bigger than if you were just holding onto the handle with your bare hand. In addition, your brain and body don't get the same feedback from gloved hands that they get from bare hands, which can make mastering proper technique and form more difficult.

To chalk or not to chalk?

Chalk is a favorite among some kettlebell users. When I competed in Girevoy Sport (GS) competitions, I always made sure the handle of my bell and my hands were really well chalked up. But, in GS, you don't put down the kettlebell for at least ten minutes, so you need all the help you can get to hang on to the kettlebell. In contrast, a typical kettlebell workout doesn't require you to hold on to the kettlebell for more than a minute or two, so chalk isn't necessary. Basically, it comes down to preference. If you have sweaty hands or if you just like to use chalk, go for it. Be aware, though, that too much chalk can actually make you get more calluses because the chalk really dries out your palms. Try using chalk for a week and then going a week without it, and see what you prefer. If you end up using chalk, make sure it's a high-quality weight lifter's chalk — the higher the quality of chalk you buy, the less likely your palms are to dry out.

Some situations do lend themselves to using tape or wearing very thin gloves on your hands. For example, you may want to do so when you have calluses that may tear or are painful to the touch. Wearing tape or thin gloves is okay to do while you're healing and still working out, but don't make it part of your regular routine because doing so can inhibit your kettlebell performance.

Safely handling the weight of your kettlebell

Besides picking out the correct size kettlebell to begin with (refer to Chapter 3), you also need to know how to safely handle the weight of the kettlebell you choose. Most of what you need to know about how to safely handle your kettlebell comes from the form and technique I help you develop for each exercise throughout this book. However, if you're ever in a position where you lose control of the kettlebell, you need to know how to safely abandon the lift. To abandon the lift, drop the kettlebell and move away from it as you do so.

Watching out for muscle strain

When beginning any new exercise routine, you need to pay careful attention to your body and make sure you don't overdo it. If you end up straining a muscle while working out, make sure to stop immediately and take the proper measures to heal yourself. Refer to Chapter 5 for solutions to minor muscle strains and soreness and for tips on what to do if you've really overdone it.

Chapter 3

Picking the Right Kettlebell and Setting Up Your Home Gym

....

....

*B*efore you can get started with your kettlebell practice, you have to choose the appropriate size weight to use. If you choose an inappropriate bell size, the benefit of the program decreases, either because the bell isn't heavy enough to yield results or because it's too heavy and results in injury. In this chapter, I provide basic flexibility and strength tests you can use to determine the right kettlebell size for you.

In addition to choosing the right size, you have to choose the right kind of kettlebell. The vast majority of the kettlebells available on the market today are a far cry from what the Russians used. Some are downright dangerous and unwieldy. Rest assured, I have tested most of what you can buy and offer my recommendations for handle type, material, and more in this chapter so that you get the best bell for your money.

You can enhance your kettlebell workouts by using other equipment, too, but you certainly don't have to spend a lot of money on exercise gadgets to get results. My recommendations for supplementary equipment in this chapter are purely optional. If your budget allows you to buy only one kettlebell, don't worry — the kettlebell's versatility, simplicity, and results will surprise you!

Finally, if you don't have room to work out at home or just like to be outside and in touch with nature, the portability of the kettlebell makes it an ideal tool for taking your workouts to the park or another venue outside your home, as you find out later in this chapter.

Testing Your Flexibility and Strength to Determine the Right Kettlebell Size

Unlike traditional weights, kettlebell exercises use your entire body to move the weight, so you can't choose your kettlebell size based on the size dumbbell (or other weight) you use. In my experience, when starting out, women typically choose a weight that's too light, and men choose one that's too heavy.

So what are good weight ranges? Women can usually start with a bell that's 14 to 18 pounds, and men can begin with a bell that's 26 to 35 pounds. (See Part IV for guidelines on choosing a kettlebell size when you're in a special situation, such as a pregnancy.) The following sections offer three basic flexibility and strength tests you can use to pinpoint the right size kettlebell for you to start with. I offer these tests as a guideline, based on my experience in teaching beginners over the years. You can find countless strength and flexibility tests out there, but I opt to keep it as simple as possible so you can begin the program right away with the right size kettlebell.

If you're a woman who can handle at least 18 pounds or a man who can handle at least 26 pounds for the vast majority of exercises in this book, you're well on your way to developing a strong and lean body. It's fine if you need to begin lighter for some exercises, especially if your upper-body strength differs greatly from your lower-body strength and you require two weights of bells. After you practice the basics, like swings (see Chapter 6) and Turkish get-ups (see Chapter 7), you'll gain a significant amount of strength quickly and be able to progress well.

The basic squat test

Ideally, you can do a rock-bottom squat (butt touching heels) while your heels stay on the floor, your torso stays upright, your knees don't cave inward, and you don't struggle to come up. However, many people can't accomplish a perfect squat before they start a kettlebell program because they never learned how to do so properly. The following instructions walk you through the *basic squat test,* which can help you assess your level of lower-body flexibility (and choose the right size kettlebell).

To do the basic squat test, follow these steps:

1. **Stand tall with your feet shoulder width apart, toes pointed out slightly, and arms out in front of you.**

2. **Slowly sit back into your hips as you reach for an imaginary chair behind you with your hips and butt; descend as low as you can without losing your form, keeping your arms straight out in front of you (see Figure 3-1).**

   For proper form, initiate the movement from your hips, rather than from your knees. Flip to Chapter 4 for more information on sitting back into your hips correctly.

   Don't let your knees come over your toes at any time when squatting.

3. **After you hit your sticking point (when you feel you can no longer descend with good form), drive through your heels and stand up tall.**

Perform five repetitions, taking note of where your form is breaking. Then write down your answers to the following questions:

1. **How low did you go in your squat without losing your form: chair height, the height of the first step on your staircase (about 8 inches), or somewhere in between?**

2. **Did your heels come off the floor during the squat movement?**

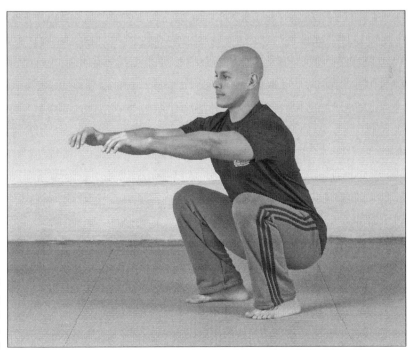

Figure 3-1:
The basic
squat test.

3. **Did your torso fall forward during the movement?**

4. **Did your knee or knees cave inward during the movement?**

5. **Did you struggle to come up?**

If you performed this squat 8 inches from the ground, or somewhere lower than chair height, and answered no to Questions 2 through 5, you can begin your lower-body movements with a kettlebell that's in the ranges I provide earlier in this chapter (14 to 18 pounds for females and 26 to 35 pounds for males). For beginners, the lower-body movements include exercises like swings (see Chapter 6), cleans (see Chapter 8), and lunges (see Chapter 10) that don't require you to bring the bell overhead.

If you performed this squat at any height listed in Question 1 but answered yes to any of Questions 2 through 5, begin your lower-body movements with a kettlebell that's in the lower range of the sizes I list earlier in this chapter (14 pounds for females and 26 pounds for males).

If you answered yes to any of Questions 2 through 5, refer to Chapter 4 for details on spine and hip essentials and Chapter 8 for tips on how to correct your squat form. Take your time figuring out how to squat correctly because proper squat form is vital to your safety in any kettlebell exercise.

The overhead squat test

While the basic squat test in the preceding section gives you a general idea of what your hip and lower-body flexibility is, the *overhead squat test* checks how mobile your upper body is and how it works together with your lower body. This test is great for assessing your shoulder and spine mobility, which you need to be aware of when choosing weight for upper-body exercises like the Turkish get-up (see Chapter 7), the press (see Chapter 8), and the snatch (see Chapter 12). Knowing how mobile you are in your shoulder and spine areas can also help you pinpoint imbalances in your body.

To do the overhead squat test, follow these steps:

1. **Stand with your feet shoulder width apart and toes pointed out slightly, and press a broomstick over your head with a wide grip (see Figure 3-2a).**

2. **Slowly sit back into your hips to descend into a squat, keeping your arms (and the stick) straight above you (see Figure 3-2b).**

   Be sure not to let the stick come forward as you squat.

3. **Drive through your heels to stand up into the start position in Step 1.**

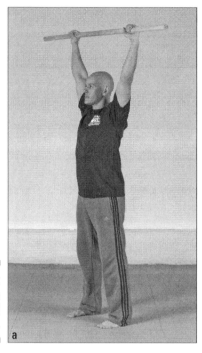 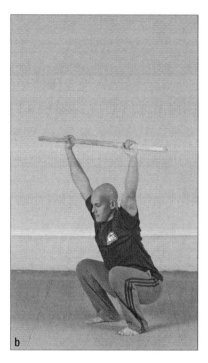

a   b

Figure 3-2:
The
overhead
squat test.

Perform five repetitions, taking note of where your form is breaking. Then write down your answers to the following questions:

1. **How low did you go in your squat without losing form: chair height, the height of the first step on your staircase (about 8 inches), or somewhere in between?**

2. **Did your arms (and the stick) fall forward during the squat movement?**

3. **Did your knee or knees cave inward during the movement?**

If you performed the overhead squat test in a low (8 inches) or rock-bottom squat and answered no to Questions 2 and 3, you possess good shoulder and spine flexibility, which means you shouldn't have any problems getting into and staying in the overhead positions of the Turkish get-up, the press, and the snatch exercises. Females in this category should use 18-pound kettlebells for overhead exercises, and men should use 26- to 35-pound bells.

The amount of flexibility you have in your upper body, coupled with your overall strength, largely determines what size kettlebell is appropriate for you to use in overhead movements. If there's a big discrepancy between your upper- and lower-body strength, you may need to buy two kettlebells, one in the lighter range for upper-body exercises and a heavier one that challenges you enough during lower-body exercises.

If you performed the overhead squat to any height from the ground but answered yes to Question 2, 3, or both, chances are you have some work to do to gain more mobility and flexibility in your spine and shoulders. Until you gain that mobility and flexibility, you need to begin with the lighter range of kettlebell sizes (14 pounds for females and 26 pounds for men) for any overhead-work-based exercises.

In some cases, a 10-pound bell for females and an 18-pound bell for males may be more appropriate. For example, you may need a lighter kettlebell if you just can't perform the overhead squat with good form or if you strain or struggle with the lighter size kettlebells (14 for women and 26 for men) when you try the overhead press test (which I describe in the next section).

The overhead press test

Unlike the preceding two tests, which focus on your flexibility, the *overhead press test* determines your strength level for overhead exercises like the Turkish get-up (see Chapter 7), the press (see Chapter 8), and the snatch (see Chapter 12). This simple test checks whether you can properly handle the size bell you're thinking about buying based on your results from the two preceding tests. You need an actual bell for this test, so, when you go to the store to buy your bell, keep the following directions handy.

To do the overhead press test, follow these steps:

1. **With the kettlebell on the ground and the handle positioned between your feet, push your hips back and bend your knees so you can reach the kettlebell with both hands; pick up the bell with both hands.**

   Use an underhand grip through the handle of the bell with your left hand and an overhand grip with your right hand to help you position the bell.

2. **Push through your heels to stand up tall; bring the bell to the left side of your chest with both hands so that the flat side of the bell rests near the left side of your chest and your left elbow is close to your rib-cage (see Figure 3-3a).**

   Pinch your glutes and abs and press your heels through the ground during this movement to stabilize the weight of the kettlebell.

3. **Release your right hand to your side, and press the bell straight overhead with control and stability (see Figure 3-3b).**

4. **Slowly bring the bell back down to the left side of your chest, and place your right hand back on top of the kettlebell handle to help you guide the bell down to the ground.**

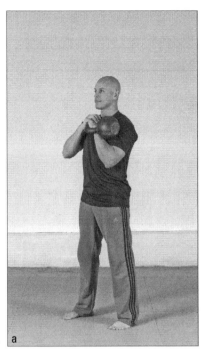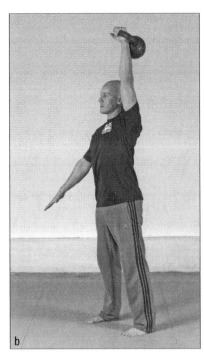

Figure 3-3:
The overhead press test.

If you pressed the bell overhead in a controlled motion — but with some resistance — chances are you've chosen a good size kettlebell to begin with for overhead exercises. If you struggled to press the bell overhead or couldn't do so at all, try the next-lower weight and repeat Steps 1 through 4.

Considering a Few Other Important Kettlebell Traits

After you determine what size kettlebell is a good starting point for you, you need to consider several other kettlebell attributes. In this section, I discuss the importance of the handle's fit and size and the kettlebell's material.

Honing in on the handle

One of the most important characteristics to look for when purchasing your kettlebell is the handle size. To get the most out of your kettlebell, carefully consider the length of the handle, the thickness of the handle, and the distance from the handle to the bell itself because these three traits have a big impact on proper performance. Here's what you need to know:

✔ **Handle length:** The handle of your kettlebell must be long enough for you to get two hands on it comfortably. If you try to put two hands on your kettlebell and your hands touch, the handle is too small. Your hands should fit on the bell with a little space in between (see Figure 3-4).

Many kettlebell exercises require the user to be able to fit two hands on the handle, so don't overlook this important trait.

✔ **Handle thickness:** If the handle is too thin or too thick, it will affect your performance. Grip the kettlebell and notice if/where your fingers meet your hand when you wrap your hand around the handle:

- If your fingers touch your palm, the handle is probably too thin.

- If your fingers are spaced more than a few inches from your palm, the handle is too thick.

The right thickness of the handle feels comfortable in your hand, and your fingers rest about 1½ inches from the heel of your palm.

If you use a handle that's too thin or thick, you risk injury because you may not be able to hold on to the bell properly for dynamic exercises, such as the swing (see Chapter 6).

✔ **Distance from handle to bell:** The distance from the handle to the bell portion of the kettlebell plays a role in how comfortable the kettlebell is in your hand, where it sits on your wrist, and, ultimately, how well you can perform with it. If the distance is too short, you can't comfortably fit your hand through the handle and it doesn't rest in the correct spot on your wrist. If the distance is too far, the kettlebell doesn't rest in the right spot on your wrist. Both instances will negatively affect your performance because you'll be uncomfortable.

A good distance from the center of the lower part of the kettlebell handle to the center of the bell portion of the kettlebell should be about 2½ inches.

The Russian Kettlebell Challenge (RKC) kettlebell is the only kettlebell on the market that's made from an original Russian kettlebell mold, which means it has the right handle size to fit both women and men perfectly (see the later section "Thinking about Quantity and Cost Before You Buy" for more information about RKC).

In addition to the handle's overall size, you need to consider the following two characteristics as you debate over which kettlebell to get:

✔ **Handle surface:** You'll risk injury and be uncomfortable if the handle surface is too smooth or too rough. A good kettlebell handle has a little bit of roughness to aid you in keeping a solid grip.

✔ **Connection between handle and bell:** It's essential that your kettlebell is made as one piece — not as two pieces with the handle attached separately. After all, you certainly don't want your kettlebell to come apart while you're swinging it over your head!

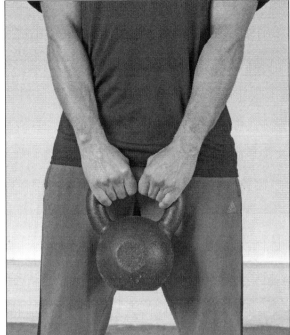

Figure 3-4:
You need to be able to fit both hands on your kettlebell's handle.

Accept no substitutions: Springing for a cast-iron bell

The original RKC kettlebell is made in one piece from cast iron, but as kettlebells became more popular, fitness manufacturers rushed to make their own versions and distinguish their kettlebells from their competitors'. The result: vinyl-coated, colored kettlebells and some bells made as two pieces (which I warn against in the preceding section).

Be wary of purchasing one of today's vinyl-coated kettlebells because several significant problems accompany them:

- ✔ Although they have visual appeal, the vinyl coating doesn't enhance performance or protect your floors; if you drop a hunk of iron, it'll damage your floor even if it has a vinyl coating on it.

- ✔ The vinyl coating doesn't have much longevity because it starts to crack and peel easily.

- ✔ Vinyl coating grabs your skin in certain positions and exercises, which can be very uncomfortable.

✔ After a kettlebell is covered with a vinyl coating, you can't see whether holes from the mold were filled with a material other than iron. If your kettlebell isn't 100-percent iron, you aren't getting the right size kettlebell that's indicated on the bell. Plus, if you're using two bells of the "same size," they may not be the same weight at all.

I recommend purchasing a kettlebell that's cast iron without a vinyl coating surrounding it. A well-made cast-iron kettlebell won't need replacing; the only risk you run is the bell collecting dust in your bedroom or rust if you leave it outside! And after all, part of the appeal of kettlebells is that they have a great history — they're the ultimate old-school fitness tool. A cast-iron bell looks much more authentic than today's vinyl-colored ones! In addition, an RKC kettlebell has been painstakingly reproduced from the Russian kettlebell, which means you can be sure the kettlebell mold is precise, the materials used are of the highest quality, and a thorough quality inspection was done before it left the factory. Making sure you buy a kettlebell that's made well and with the precision of an authentic Russian kettlebell is definitely worth the cost.

In addition to cast-iron and vinyl-coated kettlebells, you can find two other types of kettlebells in the world of fitness, although they're not worth the investment. One is an adjustable kettlebell, and the other is a sand-filled kettlebell (which you fill yourself):

✔ **Adjustable kettlebell:** An *adjustable kettlebell* doesn't perform nearly as well as a solid cast-iron bell. It's basically a series of weight plates that you add or subtract as needed. Although the idea may sound good because it supposedly helps you save space and money, an adjustable kettlebell isn't a performance-based product. It's unwieldy and doesn't distribute the weight of the bell like a solid cast-iron kettlebell. Neither trait adds anything positive to your workout routine.

Keep in mind that you won't need more than two to three sizes of kettlebells in your kettlebell practice, and they don't take up much space. Considering that one solid cast-iron kettlebell is a complete home gym, buying two or three isn't a huge investment relative to the health and fitness benefits you get from them.

✔ **Sand-filled kettlebell:** A *sand-filled kettlebell* is even worse than an adjustable kettlebell when it comes to how the weight is distributed and how it affects your performance and results. Besides having to buy a bag of sand and precisely measuring and adding it to your kettlebell, these kettlebells are typically made of plastic. Don't buy a kettlebell that's plastic unless you plan on giving it to your child to play with!

Thinking about Quantity and Cost Before You Buy

Now that you know what kind of kettlebell to buy, you need to consider a few other important things before you take out your credit card. In this section, I discuss how many kettlebells you need to get started and how much you can expect to pay for your kettlebell.

Many sporting goods retailers now sell kettlebells; you may also find them at big box retailers in the sporting goods section. If you can't find a local retailer that sells quality kettlebells and educational media, check out the original kettlebell manufacturer of the RKC kettlebell at www.russiankettlebell. com. If you buy a kettlebell online, you'll have to pay shipping, but remember, you're getting a complete home gym for a very low cost and you'll be glad you bought a higher-quality bell (although your delivery person won't be too happy about lugging a bell or two to your front door!). In addition, local RKC distributors are popping up all over the country, so check out the appendix for a distributor in your area.

How many kettlebells do you need?

As long as you take some time to determine what size kettlebell is appropriate for your strength and flexibility (by following the guidelines I provide in the "Testing Your Flexibility and Strength to Determine the Right Kettlebell Size" section), one bell is all you need to begin your kettlebell routine. However, in some cases, you may have a significant strength difference between your upper and lower body. In that case, you can use a lighter kettlebell for exercises above the shoulders and a heavier one for lower-body exercises. At most, you need to purchase two kettlebells to start your kettlebell workout program. As time goes on and you become ready to use a single heavier bell or two bells of the same size, you can still purchase relatively few pieces of equipment for a huge payoff to your health.

How much should you pay for one kettlebell?

Most kettlebells available today retail for between $30 and $47 for a 10-pound bell, $40 and $65 for a 14-pound bell, $60 and $65 for an 18-pound bell, $65 and $75 for a 26-pound bell, $70 and $80 for a 35-pound kettlebell, and up to more than $100 for the heavier sizes (in the range of 62 pounds or more). If the kettlebell is packaged with an instructional DVD from an RKC-certified instructor, rest assured you're getting a good deal.

You may think these prices are a little high for only one piece of equipment, but remember that your kettlebell is really the only piece of equipment you need — not to mention it's the only type of equipment on the market that's a cardio and weight-training program all in one. (Imagine getting rid of your treadmill and free weights and replacing them with just one kettlebell!) If you follow the instructions and programs in this book, you'll be pleasantly surprised at how versatile — and worth its price — one kettlebell really is.

Considering Other Equipment Options for Your Home Gym

Throughout this book, I suggest using several pieces of equipment other than your kettlebell to add new elements to your exercise program or to modify your program to meet your special circumstances. Know that these suggestions are completely optional — you certainly get enough of a full-body workout just by using the kettlebell. But if you want to purchase additional items, the following list is a good place to start:

- **Stopwatch or Gymboss:** Using a timing device for your workouts provides a good alternative to counting repetitions. As you become more proficient with kettlebells, doing timed sets offers you more challenge and variety than counting repetitions. If you can buy only one other item besides your kettlebell, buy a stopwatch.

- **Yoga mat:** A yoga mat is a simple, cost-effective way to create a nonslip surface in your workout area, especially if you have slippery floors.

- **Medicine ball(s):** I love incorporating heavy medicine balls into my workouts for added variety and challenge. You can start simple by substituting a kettlebell squat with a medicine ball squat, or you can add in more complex movements like a medicine ball clean and press instead of a kettlebell clean and press.

- **Jump rope:** You can use jump rope exercises as part of your warm-up or as an additional cardio element during your workout.

- **BOSU or stability ball:** You can use a BOSU or stability ball for assistance in certain exercises or simply for variety in your workout routine. (*Note:* Don't stand or kneel on either of these surfaces when using kettlebells).

- **Stretch band or strap:** A stretch band or strap is good to have for stretching after your workout, but a large towel can work just as well.

✔ **Foam roller:** I use a foam roller when I need to release really tight muscles. Although it isn't a necessity, a foam roller is a good piece of equipment to own if you're someone who doesn't have a lot of flexibility and often experiences tight muscles.

✔ **12- to 15-inch plyometric box:** Plyometric boxes can be pricey, but they're great for assisting you if you have trouble with certain kettlebell exercises, like squats. You can also use them to add explosive exercises like box jumps to your workout routine.

✔ **RKC reference material, such as DVDs and books:** A good RKC-authored book or DVD can go a long way in helping to guide your workouts and show you how to use proper technique and form. Many materials available today are focused on the beginner.

You can purchase all these additional items from your sporting goods store or online at Web sites like www.ifitnessmart.com, www.gymboss.com, and www.bosufitness.com.

Although the preceding list of equipment is optional, I recommend getting a stopwatch or Gymboss for timed workout circuits. You can purchase the other items if or when your budget allows, but keep in mind that they're in no way necessary for you to have a complete home gym.

Taking Them Bells on the Road

One thing that makes the kettlebell so convenient as an all-in-one workout tool is its portability. If you want to take your kettlebell with you, whether you're going to the gym, outside for an outdoor workout, or on a vacation or other trip, you can do so with relative ease, as you find out in this section.

Whenever you travel with your kettlebell in your car, no matter the distance, you need to secure it because an unsecured kettlebell could easily become a dangerous projectile. The easiest way to do so is to give your bell its own seat and strap the seat belt through the handle to secure it.

Taking your kettlebell to the gym

Before toting your kettlebell to the gym, you need to speak to your fitness manager. Your gym needs to have a clear, open workout area big enough that other gym patrons don't have to walk in front of, behind, or to the side of you to access their equipment. If your gym has an appropriate space, you shouldn't have a problem bringing in your own kettlebell. However, some gyms have strict policies against members bringing in their own equipment, which is why you need to check with your gym first.

Examining outdoor kettlebell workout options

If you like breathing the fresh air and sweating outside while you exercise, consider taking your kettlebell outdoors for your next workout. I love working out outside with my kettlebell, and, because I live in California, I have the benefit of almost year-round cooperative weather. But even if you live in a climate that gets only a few months of good weather, you can take advantage of it. If you have a portable device that allows you to watch workout apps, tote it along; otherwise, just take this book and your kettlebell.

Make sure you have a flat, clear area free from holes for your workout. In addition, make sure you never have to look up at the sun when doing overhead exercises like the Turkish get-up in Chapter 7 and the windmill in Chapter 10. Doing so can cause you to become disoriented and to lose control of your kettlebell, which reminds me — just because you're outside doesn't mean you should drop your bell after your sets. Always practice good technique, whether you're inside or outside. The only time dropping your kettlebell is acceptable is when you're in a precarious position and need to abandon the lift for your own safety.

With these tips in mind, take advantage of what many parks have to offer. Tools like stairs, benches, and bike paths offer variety in your workouts that you can't get at home or in the gym. In addition, many parks offer chin-up bars and other outdoor workout apparatuses that you can use in between your kettlebell exercises to add to the fun factor (monkey bars anyone?).

Going on a trip with your kettlebell

I've traveled with my kettlebell on many occasions, by both car and airplane, and you can, too. As I mention earlier in this chapter, you need to secure your kettlebell whenever you take it in a car (by strapping it in with its own seat belt). If you take it with you on a plane, you most likely have to check it as luggage (which may prompt all kinds of stares and questions). I've traveled with my kettlebell in my suitcase only once, but I think that situation was an oversight. So plan on checking your kettlebell as luggage, and, depending on how heavy it is, you may have to pay extra to do so.

After you reach your destination, take the time to find a suitable area to do your kettlebell workouts. If you're in a hotel with a gym, try doing your workout there. If you can clear an area in your room big enough to work out in, go for it. In addition, if you find a local park nearby, you can take your bell outside (weather permitting) for your workout.

Chapter 4

Moves for Success: Spine and Hip Essentials

Although good form is essential for all types of exercise, I can't emphasize enough the importance of proper back positioning and hip movement for your kettlebell workouts. By taking the time to master the spine and hip techniques in this chapter, you'll significantly decrease your chances of injury and your body will get greater benefit from the exercises:

✔ Proper spine alignment for kettlebell exercises helps your body distribute the weight of the kettlebell throughout your muscles during the movements, decreasing your chances of injury.

✔ Generating force from your hips strengthens both your back and your hips, which helps you execute the exercises with good technique (and reduces your chances of injury).

Knowing how to position your spine correctly and move from your hips when using kettlebells frees your body to access your core powerhouse; as an extra benefit, using correct form in your kettlebell exercise routine makes you stronger and more flexible in your everyday life. Just check out the essentials in this chapter to get started!

Back It Up: Getting a Grip on Neutral Spine

For most kettlebell exercises, your spine needs to be *neutral,* that is, have a natural *S* curve (just like the one in Figure 4-1). This position keeps your back safe during your workout and ensures that you reap the full benefits of your kettlebell routine.

Getting into a neutral spine position is quite simple and natural. The majority of students I've worked with can get into it easily, and the good news is that you'll know exactly when you have it. Try this little exercise: Grab your desk chair and sit down. Chances are you just sat down, initiating the movement from your knees. Now, stand back up, take a step forward, think about reaching your butt back to sit down, and pause before you do. Notice anything different? If you do this exercise correctly, you notice a natural *S* curve in your back as you reach back for the chair, first with your butt and hips, letting your knees follow their lead.

In the following sections, I provide two more easy neutral spine exercises to practice — just to make sure you get it right before you pick up your kettlebell. I also explain the importance of keeping a flat back (and avoiding a rounded back) during your movements, and I show you the proper head and neck position for a neutral spine.

I'm sure you've heard the advice to lift with your legs and not with your back, but you may not always heed that advice. Lucky for you, this section teaches you how to keep your spine neutral and initiate your movement from the hips to prevent injury. It makes the lift-with-your-legs advice a natural movement, so you'll never again lift with your back when you pick up something — a kettlebell or anything else.

Figure 4-1:
The natural
S curve of
a neutral
spine.

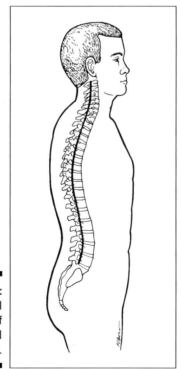

Sitting back to achieve neutral spine

The term *sitting back into your hips* may not sound familiar to you, but I use it throughout this book when referring to properly starting many of the kettlebell exercises. As you practice how to sit back into your hips to achieve neutral spine in the following exercises, the movement will likely feel natural if you're fairly flexible and have reasonable strength. But don't despair if you feel like you're going to fall on your butt. Figuring out how to sit back into your hips increases your mobility and strength rather quickly, and it won't be long before the movement feels natural for your body.

In this section, I focus on two simple exercises — the box squat and the face-the-wall squat — to help you achieve neutral spine by sitting back into your hips. Throughout the book, I also refer to these two exercises as corrective techniques for when you have difficulty with a particular exercise. You may want to dog-ear these sections, in case you need to refer to them later.

The box squat

The *box squat* is a very simple exercise that I want you to try first thing to help you assess how well you achieve neutral spine and identify where you need some practice before you start using your kettlebell. To do this exercise, you need a sturdy plyometric box or a chair that's about 18 inches tall.

To do the box squat, follow these steps:

1. **Place your box or chair directly behind you, take one full step forward, and stand with your feet shoulder width apart and your arms straight out in front of you.**

2. **Look at a focal point on the ground 6 feet in front of you, hold your arms straight out in front of you, put your weight in your heels, and reach back for the box or chair by initiating the movement from your hips, letting your knees follow your hips' lead (see Figure 4-2); continue to reach back until you lightly tap the box or chair with your butt.**

   Your spine will be in neutral position as long as your hips move before your knees do.

   Think about reaching back for an imaginary wall with your hips while you keep your weight in your heels.

3. **Drive through your heels to stand up tall to your start position, squeezing your glutes and abs as you do so.**

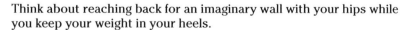

Perform ten repetitions, making sure to reposition yourself after each rep as needed so that you're reaching back sufficiently for the chair with each rep.

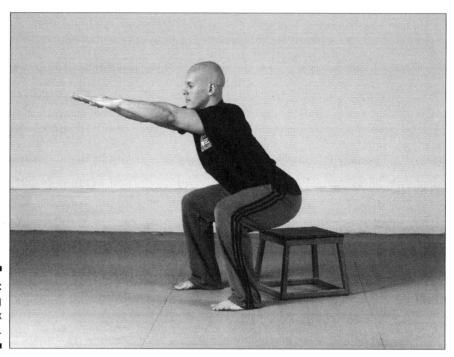

Figure 4-2:
Performing
the box
squat.

At the Russian Kettlebell Challenge (RKC) certification course, students partner with each other for this exercise. One student gets on his hands and knees to form a "box" with his body; the other student reaches back toward the "box" (but doesn't sit down) to practice the technique. If you don't have a plyometric box or a chair that's 18 inches tall, find a willing partner to help you do this exercise. Just remember not to actually sit back on your partner!

After performing your practice repetitions, take note of your movement patterns. Ask yourself the following questions to assess how you're doing:

- ✔ Can you keep your weight in your heels throughout the movement without feeling like you're going to fall back?
- ✔ Are you reaching back with your hips first and then flexing your knees to follow your hips' lead?
- ✔ Do you feel (or see) a natural curve in your spine as you sit back?

If you answer yes to all the preceding questions, you're ready to practice the face-the-wall squat in the next section. If you answer no to any of the questions, take more time to practice the box squat until you can answer yes to all the questions. Then you can move to the face-the-wall squat.

The face-the-wall squat

The *face-the-wall squat* is simple to do; the only equipment you need is a clutter-free wall space about the length of your arm span. Like the box squat, this squat helps you achieve neutral spine and clues you in to areas where your technique may need some work before you start using your kettlebell.

To do the face-the-wall squat, follow these steps:

1. **Face the wall with your feet shoulder width apart, and stand about 6 to 10 inches from the wall with your arms down at your side; put your weight into your heels.**

2. **Keep facing forward with your eyes fixed on the wall (not looking up) as you push your hips back behind you, letting your knees bend; pull yourself down to about 90 degrees, keeping your arms at your side (see Figure 4-3).**

   As in the box squat, your spine will be in neutral position as long as your spine has a natural *S* curve and your hips move before your knees do.

3. **After you reach the bottom position, drive through your heels to stand up tall to your start position, tightening your abs and glutes as you do so.**

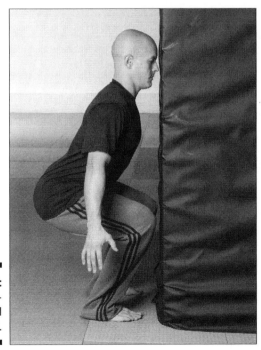

Figure 4-3:
The face-the-wall squat.

Perform ten repetitions. After you perform your practice repetitions, use the three questions from the previous box squat section to assess yourself. If you answer yes to all three questions, you probably won't have any problems getting into neutral spine for kettlebell exercises. If you answer no to any of the questions, take some more time to practice the face-the-wall squat (and the box squat, too, if you want extra practice).

If you find yourself turning your head to one side while doing the face-the-wall squat, adjust your positioning so that you aren't so close to the wall. But don't move back too far because doing so won't assist you in getting into the neutral spine position. After all, your back automatically gets into neutral spine position when you're close enough to the wall and facing it.

Understanding the importance of maintaining a neutral spine

When starting and finishing all kettlebell exercises, you absolutely must know the difference between a rounded (vertebral flexion) back and a neutral back:

- ✔ A *rounded back* looks like a hunched back and happens when you round your shoulders toward the ground as you initiate your movement; it can either be slight or exaggerated (see Figure 4-4a).

- ✔ A neutral back is when you have a subtle natural *S* curve in your back as you initiate your movement from your hips (see Figure 4-4b). It doesn't feel exaggerated or forced; it feels natural.

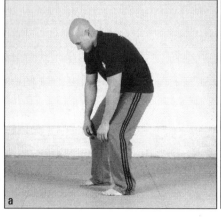
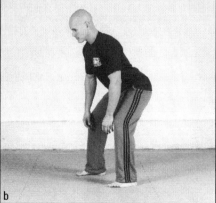

Figure 4-4: A rounded back versus a neutral back.

a

b

When using kettlebells (or lifting anything, in general), make sure you don't round your back at any point during your exercises (and that includes picking up and setting down the kettlebell!). Doing so puts your back in an unstable position, which makes it vulnerable to injury. Maintaining a neutral spine, on the other hand, creates a stable base by helping you activate your core and other major muscle groups, which you then use to lift your kettlebell. So be aware of how you start and finish each exercise, as well as how you perform the steps in between; having perfect form throughout the exercise will lessen your chance of injury and get you the best results. Keep your spine neutral, and initiate your movement only from the hip and knee joints (see the "It's All in the Hips" section for more details on how to move your hips properly).

Keep practicing the box squat and the face-the-wall squat until you can easily get into neutral spine. These exercises are the simplest ways to practice getting into — and staying in — the right position for your kettlebell exercises.

Positioning your head and neck properly

The term *neutral spine* relates to more than just your back position; it also describes your head and neck position. You want to position your head and neck correctly so you don't put any stress or pressure on them (or your spine), which could lead to injury. Maintaining the right head and neck position is easy to do if you find a focal point that's approximately 6 feet in front of you on the floor (see Figure 4-5). Don't look straight down or straight ahead.

By fixing your eyes on a focal point 6 feet away and down throughout any kettlebell exercise (including its start and finish), you keep your head and neck in alignment with your spine. As a result, you won't experience any strain or stress in your neck or back.

Figure 4-5:
The proper head and neck position in neutral spine.

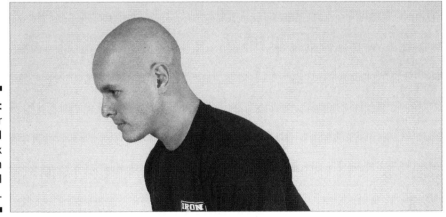

Take a moment to practice getting into neutral spine with the help of the exercises I describe earlier in this chapter, and focus your eyes 6 feet in front of you on the floor. To help you remember to maintain good head and neck position throughout your workouts, you can use tape or some other marking device to make a focal point on the floor of your workout area.

It's All in the Hips

If you usually do traditional weight lifting or use machines for your workouts, chances are you don't move and use much of your hip power when exercising because most traditional exercises don't show you how to move and access your hips. In fact, many traditional exercises make your hips less mobile.

Working out with kettlebells, on the other hand, offers you a completely different perspective on what it means to move and use your entire body (including your hips). With kettlebells, much of your movement originates from the hips. Although this concept may sound strange at first, moving from your hips and fully engaging your core when exercising feels quite natural after you've practiced for a while.

Just by looking at the hips (you know, the ball-and-socket joints between your pelvis and upper-leg bones), you may not think they're a powerhouse for your body, but strong hips make activities like standing and walking effortless (see Figure 4-6 for an illustration of the hip bones). If you don't have strong hips, your body has to use other areas of the body a lot more, which can lead to painful back or knee problems. For this reason, strong and mobile hips may just be the most important benefit your kettlebell exercises give you.

The power that you're able to generate from your hips (in other words, your *hip snap*) largely determines how much weight you can handle when using kettlebells and what kind of results you get from the exercises. When you're beginning a kettlebell program, you start with a certain size kettlebell (see Chapter 3 for details on determining which size is right for you). As time goes on, you'll likely want to progress to a heavier bell. Before you do so, however, make sure you master the hip snap basics that I cover in the following sections so you can progress safely to a heavier kettlebell. After all, a kettlebell that's too light really doesn't do much for the average healthy individual. To benefit from strength training, your body needs to be challenged and taxed during your workout. And to challenge your body safely with kettlebells, you need to have a strong and powerful hip snap.

Practice your hip snap with every repetition and during every workout. Each snap should be intentional and deliberate — no matter what size kettlebell you're using. The amount of force and tension you create while using the kettlebell makes all the difference between benefiting from the program and getting lackluster results. Also, if you don't use your hips to move the bell, your body has to use more of other areas of your body — using your biceps to clean the bell, for example (see Chapter 8 to figure out what I'm talking about) — which causes you not only to risk injury but also to cheat yourself out of developing strong and mobile hips and a powerful core.

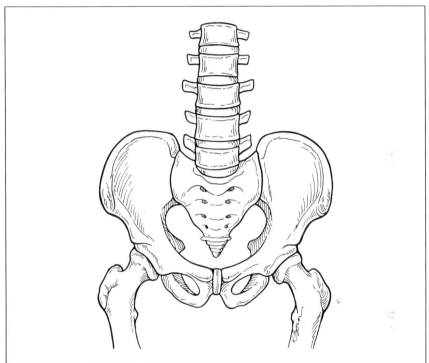

Figure 4-6:
The anatomy of the hips.

Finding the perfect hip snap stance

Before you can learn the hip snap, you need to get yourself into the right start position. A good hip snap requires you to be able to sit back far enough into your hips that you can access your core's powerhouse of muscles. If your feet are positioned too far apart or too close together, you won't be able to do the hip snap properly, so be sure to follow the steps in this section carefully.

Make sure the handle of your kettlebell isn't too wide. If it is, it'll force you to have a wider stance because, if you get into the proper stance, the overly wide handle will rub up against your inner thighs, causing you a lot of discomfort. That discomfort, in turn, will impede how far back you can sit into your hips, which will negatively affect your hip snap. (Refer to Chapter 3 for picking the right kettlebell.) Although little nuances like this one seem trivial, they're important and will affect your performance and progress.

Getting into the perfect hip snap stance is different for everyone because everyone's body is built differently. However, this section gives you a few general guidelines to follow to help you find your stance. As you begin to use kettlebells in your regular workout routine, you can adjust your stance as needed. Follow these steps to find your perfect hip snap stance:

1. **Stand tall with your feet shoulder width apart, toes pointing forward, and abs and glutes tight.**

2. **Sit back with your hips as you did in the box squat that I describe earlier in this chapter (see the section "The box squat").**

3. **Drive through your heels to stand back up tall.**

4. **Widen your stance slightly (a couple of inches), and repeat Steps 2 and 3 until you find your perfect hip snap stance.**

Most likely, this slightly wider stance is what I mean when I say, "Find your perfect hip snap stance." Your feet are slightly wider than shoulder width apart, you can reach back into your hips without feeling like you're going to fall backward, and a kettlebell fits well enough between your legs (the handle of your kettlebell shouldn't rub against your inner thighs, but your forearms will).

Rooting yourself for a strong hip snap

After you find the right stance, rooting yourself into the ground is the next essential step to acquiring a strong and powerful hip snap. *Rooting yourself* simply means planting your weight into the ground so that you're able to remain solid and steady throughout the kettlebell exercises. In other words, the kettlebell should never shift your weight either backward or forward during exercise. But unless you properly establish your footing before you pick up the kettlebell, it will do just that.

Make sure you're barefoot or wearing very flat-soled sneakers (like boxing shoes) when working out with kettlebells. Doing so allows you to feel the ground and properly root yourself for a strong hip snap.

To root yourself in preparation for the hip snap, follow these steps:

1. **Get into your perfect hip snap stance by following Steps 1 through 4 in the "Finding the perfect hip snap stance" section.**

2. **To ground yourself, stomp your left foot into the ground and then stomp your right foot into the ground, pressing your heels into the ground and gripping the floor with your toes.**

You should feel grounded in this position, and, if someone tried to knock you back or push you over, she should have a difficult time doing so.

When you stomp your feet into the ground, do so deliberately. If you merely step your feet, your brain won't get the same type of feedback from the ground that it gets when you stomp.

Generating force from the ground up and snapping your hips

Using the proper hip snap movement throughout your kettlebell routine makes your entire body strong and powerful. When you practice a hip snap, think about driving through your heels and imagine the force you generate moving up your body and out through the top of your head.

Because some students have difficulty mastering the hip snap while using a kettlebell, I suggest that you practice the following technique without your kettlebell. When you're ready to pick up the kettlebell, move on to the section "Connecting with your kettlebell as you snap your hips." As you start practicing the exercises in the rest of this book, refer back to this section whenever you need help with snapping your hips and generating force.

All too often, new students confuse the kettlebell hip snap with a pelvic tilt. Doing so limits how much force you can generate because you wait too long to snap your hips and simply end up doing a pelvic tilt to move the kettlebell (instead of generating force from the ground up with the hip snap). Not only is this form incorrect, but it also will eventually lead to injury. Follow the steps in this section carefully to make sure you generate force from the ground up and snap your hips rather than tilt your pelvis.

To generate force from the ground up and snap your hips, follow these steps:

1. **Get into your perfect hip snap stance (which you establish earlier in the "Finding the perfect hip snap stance" section), and then root yourself into the ground.**

   See the "Rooting yourself for a strong hip snap" section for details on how to root yourself properly.

2. **With your arms out in front of you, reach back with your hips for an imaginary box, chair, or wall (until you really feel your butt reaching back and your weight in your heels), keeping a neutral spine (see Figure 4-7a).**

   Check out the "Back It Up: Getting a Grip on Neutral Spine" section for tips on how to maintain a neutral spine throughout your exercises.

3. **Drive through your heels, lock out your knees, and tighten your abs and glutes as you snap your hips forward (see Figure 4-7b), and return to a standing position with a tall spine.**

   The hip snap that I describe here is powerful; it begins when you drive through your heels and continues as you lock out your knees, tighten your thighs, glutes, and abs, and stand tall with all your muscles tight at the top. It's a forceful, deliberate movement that uses the power you generate from your core to move the kettlebell. You're not simply tucking your butt under your hips or pushing your hips forward at the top of the movement.

   Don't hyperextend your back when you snap your hips to come back to standing. In the top position, your spine should be tall and your body should resemble a vertical line without any significant leaning back.

Perform ten repetitions to feel comfortable with the hip snap.

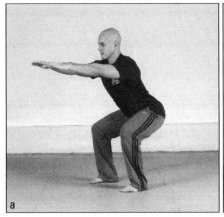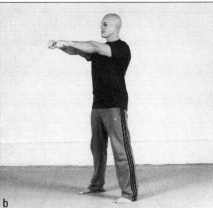

Figure 4-7:
The hip
snap.

Connecting with your kettlebell as you snap your hips

When you're ready to pick up your kettlebell for the basic exercises in Part II of this book, you need to make sure your body fully accesses its hip power to move the kettlebell (otherwise, you may injure whatever other part of your body you use to move the bell). Lucky for you, this section is here to help you make a few adjustments that allow you to access the hip power you need to build strength (and avoid injury) in your kettlebell routine.

As you begin practicing your hip snap with the kettlebell, be sure to do the following to help your body access its maximum hip power and avoid injury:

- ✔ Use a kettlebell that isn't too light or too heavy.
- ✔ Maintain a connection to the kettlebell (in other words, don't let the bell get ahead of you).

You know you've chosen a kettlebell that's too light when it flops around in the top position of the exercise or when the exercise just doesn't feel challenging enough. Your bell's too heavy when you feel yourself straining under the weight at any time during your exercise. If you've chosen the wrong size kettlebell, turn to Chapter 3 to find out how to pick the right size.

If you're letting your kettlebell get ahead of you (and, thus, aren't staying connected to your bell), try doing the corrective technique in this section to fix your hip snap. After all, if you stay connected to your kettlebell during all your exercises, the timing for all your movements is perfect, which keeps the timing of your hip snap on target and your hips engaged. As a result, your movements become fluid and graceful, and you don't have to force anything even though your body is working hard to move the kettlebell. Even if you didn't pick the perfect size kettlebell the first time, the corrective technique in this section can help you get the timing of your hip snap precise enough to move through the exercises in this book with confidence.

Staying connected to your kettlebell may sound a little Zen, but maintaining this kind of visualization really does improve your hip snap form. You don't necessarily need to "be one" with your kettlebell, but not letting it get too far out in front of you is the difference between having good form and having sloppy form.

To practice staying connected with your kettlebell (and, in turn, improving your overall technique), follow these steps:

1. **Stand in your perfect hip snap stance, and then root yourself into the ground.**

   Check out the section "Finding the perfect hip snap stance" for more about how to get into the right stance and the section "Rooting yourself for a strong hip snap" for more details on how to root yourself properly.

2. **Straighten both your arms out in front of you at about chest height.**

3. **Bring your straightened arms down toward your rib cage, and, as you connect your arms to your rib cage, sit back into your hips (see Figure 4-8).**

   To find out how to sit back into your hips the right way, turn to the earlier sections "The box squat" and "The face-the-wall squat."

4. **Drive through your heels to stand back up; as you do, let your hips bump your arms up to chest height so that your arms just float up.**

   In other words, keep your arms connected to your rib cage until the moment when you snap your hips, at which time your arms briefly leave your rib cage (a movement that your hip snap initiates).

Perform ten repetitions to feel comfortable with this movement. Practicing how the movement should feel before you start using your kettlebell programs your body to do the movement properly so that staying connected to your kettlebell is an automatic body response when you pick up the bell.

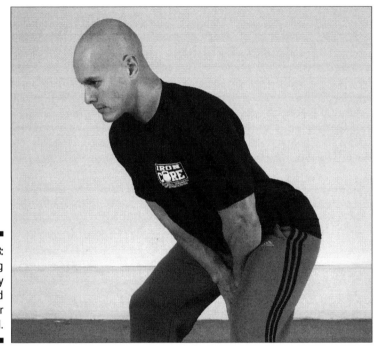

Figure 4-8:
Practicing how to stay connected to your kettlebell.

Chapter 5

Breathing Right, Warming Up, Cooling Down, and Taking Care

* *

In This Chapter

▶ Figuring out how to breathe properly during a workout

▶ Warming up and cooling down with ease

▶ Caring for yourself if you're sore (or worse)

▶ Challenging yourself with active rest options

* *

So you've bought a kettlebell, set up your home gym, and mastered the essential spine and hip movements. But wait! You're not quite ready to dive into a kettlebell routine; before you begin, you need to discover this chapter's basics on breathing right, warming up, cooling down, and taking care of yourself:

✔ All too often new kettlebell students don't want to hear themselves breathing during their workouts, but deliberate, deep inhalation and forceful exhalation during kettlebell movements is important. How and when you breathe during your kettlebell workouts is paramount to getting good results and preventing injuries. Precise breathing and breath control works to protect your core while you're slinging around the kettlebell.

✔ Although you may be ready to dive right in to the main event, warming up is an important component to your kettlebell workouts. You don't have to spend much time doing so because the warm-up exercises I describe in this chapter are designed to prepare your body quickly for kettlebell exercise. The best warm-up options are movements that mimic your kettlebell exercise routine.

✔ Although you may be inclined to collapse on the floor or bend over to catch your breath after you finish your kettlebell exercises, you need to cool down your body immediately after you finish your routine. The best cool-down routines bring your heart rate down slowly — they can be as simple as walking around after your workout and then doing two to three of the cool-down options I describe in this chapter.

✔ Determining when you've overdone it either during or after your workouts is one key to keeping your body and mind healthy for the long haul. I offer suggestions on how to decide whether your muscles are just sore because your workout was intense or you've really hurt yourself by pushing too hard. Either way, I give you some quick and easy solutions to get you back on track.

And don't forget: After you've been doing kettlebells for a while, you can challenge yourself with some extra moves called active rest options; I give you the scoop at the end of this chapter.

Breathing Properly

Perhaps you work out at a gym that prohibits grunting — I've seen signs posted on the walls of mainstream gyms prohibiting loud grunting or breathing. I can understand the management's motivation to keep the club atmosphere quiet. However, holding your breath or not breathing properly during kettlebells (or any weight-training exercise) can be dangerous. So, if you've been taught to be quiet during your workouts, forget that philosophy now! And even though the people you live with may wonder what all the noise is while you're working out, breathing properly helps you get the best possible results from your kettlebell program. Not only will you stay off the injured list, but your abs will feel the burn and any belly fat you have will begin to melt away. Read on to find out how to breathe properly for maximum results.

Understanding how to relax under tension

When it comes to kettlebell workouts, a very important distinction exists between tension and relaxation. By no means do you want to relax your whole body while executing a kettlebell exercise. But, at the same time, you don't want to hold so much tension during your workouts that you can't breathe properly or give your muscles the chance to get stronger and more flexible. You must be able to relax under tension at certain times while executing kettlebell exercises. Although this concept may seem like an oxymoron, relaxing under tension is possible.

The easiest way to relax under tension is to relax your facial muscles while executing an exercise. Although kettlebell workouts are intense and your face will show it at times, try to be conscious of how much tension is showing on your face and try to relax your facial muscles. Doing so helps regulate how much tension you keep in the rest of your body and helps you breathe fully and properly.

Tightening your virtual belt with diaphragmatic breathing

You may think of breathing as something you do automatically; you probably aren't conscious of how you breathe. The majority of people breathe with shallow, chest-and-shoulder breaths, but breathing this way doesn't give you the full benefit that transporting oxygen completely in and out of your body gives you. A breath should be deliberate and deep and use your diaphragm rather than your chest (hence, the term *diaphragmatic breathing*).

Diaphragmatic breathing is a type of breathing that allows you to tighten your virtual belt, an action called *abdominal bracing*. Using diaphragmatic breathing to brace your abs helps you protect your core (spine included) from the weight and force of the kettlebell by stabilizing your core with breath control. It also allows your body to get oxygen in and out properly. Abdominal bracing is a technique that martial artists, fighters, and boxers know well, and it's a great technique for you to use during your kettlebell workouts.

When you brace your abdominals, imagine that you're bracing your core (rib cage to pelvis) for a punch, but don't hold your breath; you need to continue to breathe throughout any exercise you're performing.

Taking the time to figure out how to breathe using the diaphragmatic breathing technique will not only improve your workout results but also help you stay focused with each repetition. Try this simple exercise to figure out how to breathe using your diaphragm:

1. **Lie on your back on the floor, and put one hand on your chest and one hand on your stomach (see Figure 5-1).**

2. **Take a deep and deliberate inhale through your nose, keeping your lips tight or pursed.**

   As you inhale through your nose, you should see and feel only your stomach expand and fill with air.

3. **Exhale, putting your tongue behind your teeth and forcing the air out of your stomach to make an audible sound.**

   Your lips can be in a "smile" position as you exhale (refer to Figure 5-1). The sound you make during your exhale should mimic the sound that letting the air out of a tire makes (an audible *ssss* sound).

Repeat the exercise for ten breaths.

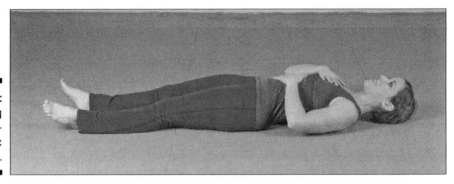

Figure 5-1:
Practicing
diaphrag-
matic
breathing.

You may feel a bit dizzy after practicing a few reps of the diaphragmatic breathing exercise. If you do, stop the exercise and try again later in the day. It may take you a while to work up to ten diaphragmatic breaths, especially if you're a shallow chest breather.

Diaphragmatic breathing enables you to have the best-possible core stabilization when using kettlebells, so practice it until it becomes natural. But always be mindful of how and when you're breathing while executing kettlebell exercises.

Knowing when to inhale and exhale during your kettlebell exercises

After you understand the concepts of relaxing under tension and abdominal bracing, you need to apply that knowledge to your kettlebell practice.

In general, you want to inhale when you lift the kettlebell from the ground and exhale as you execute the lift. Although your breathing will vary slightly depending on the exercise you're doing, when in doubt, you can safely follow this guideline.

The following list outlines how to breathe for four basic kettlebell movements. After you understand the breathing patterns for these basic exercises, breathing properly during the other exercises will come naturally.

- ✔ **How to breathe for the swing (see Chapter 6):** Breathing during the swing is easy. Take a diaphragmatic inhale as you pick up the kettlebell and bring it behind you; forcefully exhale (making an audible *ssss* sound) as you bring the kettlebell from the back swing position to the top position. As the kettlebell is descending from the top position, take another diaphragmatic inhale. Repeat this process as you continue with the swing.

- ✔ **How to breathe for the clean (see Chapter 8):** Take a diaphragmatic inhale as you pick up the kettlebell; exhale as you bring the bell into the rack position. Before returning the kettlebell to the floor or back swing position, fill your stomach with air by taking another deep, diaphragmatic inhale. Repeat this process as you continue with the clean.

✔ **How to breathe for the squat (see Chapter 8):** Like you do for the clean, take a diaphragmatic inhale as you pick up the kettlebell; then exhale as you bring the bell into the rack position. When the kettlebell is in the rack position, take a deep, diaphragmatic inhale as you descend into the squat position. As you drive through your heels to stand up tall, forcefully exhale (making an audible *ssss* sound). Repeat this process as you continue with the squat.

✔ **How to breathe for the press (see Chapter 8):** Like you do for the clean and the squat, take a diaphragmatic inhale as you pick up the kettlebell; then exhale as you bring the bell into the rack position. Before you press the kettlebell from the rack position to the overhead position, take a deep, diaphragmatic inhale; as you press, exhale forcefully (making an audible *ssss* sound) to help you get the bell into the top, lockout position. From the top position, inhale as you bring the bell back down into the rack position. Repeat this process as you continue with the press.

Don't ever hold your breath! As you soon as you take your deep inhale, you need to push or force the air back out. At no time during your workout should you hold your breath.

Off to a Good Start: Warming Up

Because kettlebell exercises truly mimic your everyday movements, you don't have to do as much to safely prepare your body for the exercises as you'd have to do for exercises that focus on isolated muscle groups. (I have to admit: I don't spend too much time warming up for my kettlebell workouts. In fact, I may do only two or three warm-up options from the following sections before I begin my kettlebell routine.)

The best options for warming up for your kettlebell exercises are the dynamic movements, kettlebell warm-up options, and Z-Health options that I describe in the following sections. To get started, you can choose one from each category; then, as you progress in your kettlebell practice, pick the warm-ups you like best and the ones your body responds to the most.

Doing dynamic stretches

Dynamic stretches are a quick and effective way to prepare your body for exercise; they mimic your everyday movements as well as the movements you do with your kettlebell during your workout. I provide three dynamic warm-up stretches in the following sections.

The body weight squat

The *body weight squat* is an effective, quick warm-up that's also easy to do. It warms up your lower body and really gets you moving for your kettlebell workouts. To do this exercise, follow these steps:

1. **Stand with your feet shoulder width apart or slightly wider than shoulder width.**

2. **Keep your weight on your heels and push back into your hips as your arms come out in front of you (see Figure 5-2); slowly pull yourself down as far as you can go comfortably while keeping your heels on the ground.**

3. **After you hit your lowest point, drive through your heels and come back to standing.**

Perform ten repetitions without resting in between them.

The downward dog to cobra (or pumps)

This warm-up exercise borrows the downward dog and cobra poses from yoga. In kettlebell class, these two poses together are called *pumps*. If you only have time to warm up with one exercise, this one would be at the top of my list. Pumps warm up your body from top to bottom rather quickly.

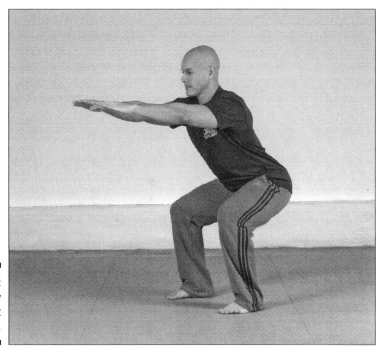

Figure 5-2: The body weight squat.

To do this exercise, follow these steps:

1. **Stand with your feet shoulder width apart and slowly bend at the waist to bring your hands to the floor in front of you, bending your knees if you need to.**

2. **Walk your hands out in front of you until your body is in the shape of an inverted *V* (called pike position).**

3. **Try to press your heels into the ground as you press your hands into the floor, as if you're pushing the floor away from you, keeping your hips pointed up toward the ceiling (see Figure 5-3a).**

   You're now in the downward dog position.

4. **Slowly bring your hips toward the ground as you bring your chest and head up toward the ceiling; keep your glutes pinched (see Figure 5-3b).**

   You're now in the cobra position.

5. **Push back up into the downward dog position I describe in Step 3.**

Figure 5-3:
The
downward
dog to
cobra.

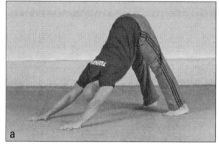 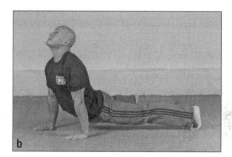

Perform ten repetitions without resting in between them.

The push-up to T-hold

The *push-up to T-hold* is the most difficult dynamic warm-up I describe in this chapter because the movement requires a tremendous amount of core strength to execute it properly. To do this exercise, follow these steps:

1. **Get into the plank position, with your arms shoulder width apart, your shoulders positioned over your wrists, your palms flat on the ground, and your elbows close to your rib cage.**

2. **Keeping your core, glutes, and thighs tight, let your elbows bend (but keep them close to your rib cage) as you slowly lower yourself about**

2 to 6 inches from the ground; then push back up to the start position and continue with Step 3.

If you aren't good at push-ups (which is what you're doing in Steps 1 and 2), you can do the push-up on your knees and then reposition yourself when you get to the *T* position in Step 3.

3. **From the top of the push-up position, lift your right hand as you rotate your body to the right, keeping your weight on your left side and bringing your right arm above you to form a *T*; stack your right foot on your left foot and look straight ahead of you (see Figure 5-4).**

4. **Hold this *T* pose for five to ten seconds, keeping your core and glutes tight.**

5. **Return to the plank position I describe in Step 1.**

Perform a total of four repetitions (two on each side) without resting in between them.

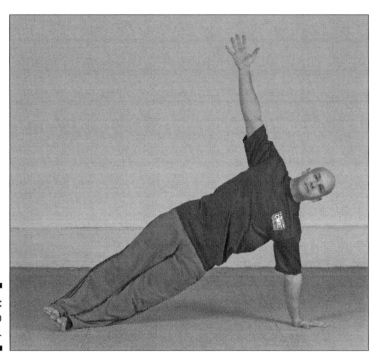

Figure 5-4: The push-up to T-hold.

Incorporating your kettlebell in your warm-up

Some kettlebell exercises, such as the Turkish get-up (see Chapter 7) and the windmill (see Chapter 10), can double as excellent dynamic warm-up options, but they require time to master their form and technique. So, to help you get started right away, this section looks at a few other less-involved warm-up options that use the kettlebell.

The warm-ups using the kettlebell are perfect if you're short on time or just can't wait to pick up your kettlebell! They warm up your body, getting it ready for your workout, and build strength at the same time.

The halo

The *halo* packs a powerful punch into one warm-up exercise. If you're using a challenging-enough size kettlebell, this exercise helps you warm up your upper body quickly and also works your abdominals. It's a great core-strengthening exercise that takes only about 30 seconds to 1 minute of work to feel the burn.

To do this exercise, follow these steps:

1. **Stand with your feet shoulder width apart, and hold the kettlebell upside down by the handle with both hands positioned at chest level (so the flat part of the bell is facing up); pinch your glutes and abs, and drive your heels into the ground.**

   As you hold the kettlebell by the handle, make sure your arms are bent and close to your sides.

2. **Bring the kettlebell up and rotate it to the right around your head toward the back of your neck so the flat part of the bell is facing down (see Figure 5-5a); continue to move the kettlebell around your head until it's back at the start position in Step 1.**

   Keep your elbows bent and parallel to each other as you move the kettlebell.

3. **Continue to circle the kettlebell around your head to the right, keeping your elbows close to your head throughout the movement (see Figure 5-5b).**

Trace a "halo" around your head to the right for 15 repetitions; then switch directions and repeat for 15 repetitions. Perform two sets total.

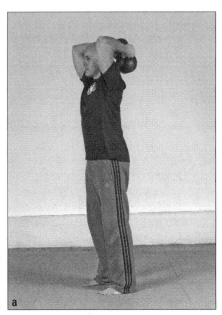 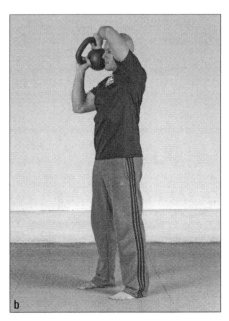

Figure 5-5:
The halo.

a   b

The overhead hold

The *overhead hold* is an effective core and upper-body warm-up; it also reminds you how to keep your shoulders in their sockets when executing exercises like the military press and the snatch (see Chapter 8 for more details about the military press and Chapter 12 for more about the snatch).

To do the overhead hold, follow these steps:

1. **Stand with your feet shoulder width apart, and bring the kettlebell into the rack position on the left side by pushing your hips back and letting your knees bend so that you can put your left hand through the handle of the kettlebell with an underhand grip; place your right hand in an overhand grip over your left to assist you in bringing the kettlebell (which is facing sideways) into the rack position.**

   See Chapter 8 for more details on how to achieve the rack position.

2. **Press the kettlebell up overhead into full lockout position with your left arm straight and your left bicep in line with your ear (see Figure 5-6); hold this position for 20 seconds.**

   Drop your right arm to your side as you hold the kettlebell with your left hand.

3. **Bring the kettlebell back into the rack position on your left side.**

Perform four reps (two on each side).

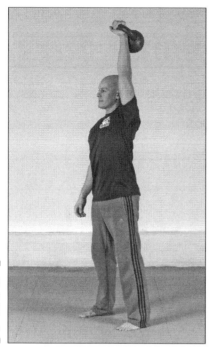

Figure 5-6:
The
overhead
hold.

If you can't keep your elbow locked and your shoulder sunken in the socket, down, and away from your ear when executing this exercise, you need to work on your shoulder and thoracic flexibility before you can do this movement safely. Practice the half Turkish get-up with a light weight (see Chapter 7); as your stability and flexibility increase, you can progress to the full Turkish get-up in Chapter 7 and then back to the overhead hold position I discuss here.

For a little variety and more of a challenge, perform the overhead hold with two kettlebells of the same size. In this advanced variation, one rep works out both arms rather than just one as the original exercise does.

After you perform the overhead hold with either one or two kettlebells, try walking around for 20 seconds as you hold the bell(s) instead of standing still. Make sure to keep your glutes and core engaged while you walk. By walking around with the kettlebells overhead, you gain even more stability in your shoulders and core than you do with the stationary overhead hold.

The farmer's hold and farmer's walk

The *farmer's hold* and *farmer's walk* not only warm up the entire body quickly but also strengthen your grip on the kettlebell. Having a strong grip and building its endurance are important parts of your kettlebell training, especially during long sets or sets during which you use a heavy kettlebell.

To do the farmer's hold, follow these steps:

1. **Stand with your feet shoulder width apart and your glutes, thighs, and abs tight; hold the kettlebell by the handle in your left hand with your arm down by your side (see Figure 5-7).**

2. **Concentrate on driving through your heels and keeping your abs, glutes, and thighs tight, and squeeze the handle of the kettlebell as you hold the position for one minute without setting the kettlebell down.**

Perform four reps (two on each side).

To perform the farmer's walk, follow the instructions for the farmer's hold, but instead of standing still, walk for one minute either forward or in a large circle with your kettlebell as you maintain the farmer's hold position on the left side. Then switch sides and walk for one minute as you complete the farmer's hold on the right side.

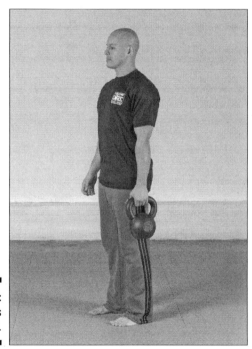

Figure 5-7:
The farmer's
hold.

Keep good posture during both the farmer's hold and the farmer's walk by keeping your abs and glutes engaged and your shoulders lowered into your lat muscles (which, in general, run under your shoulders, behind your arms, and down your back).

The waiter's hold and waiter's walk

The *waiter's hold* and *waiter's walk* are variations of the farmer's walk; they require you to have two kettlebells of the same size so that you can work both sides of your body at the same time. Just follow these steps for the waiter's hold:

1. **Stand with your feet together, keeping your glutes, thighs, and abs tight; hold one kettlebell by the handle down at your right side and the other bell down at your left side.**

2. **Bring the kettlebell on your left side into rack position by pushing your hips back, letting your knees bend, and bringing the kettlebell snug up to your chest with the thumb of your left hand touching your collarbone; pull your left elbow into your rib cage.**

    Hold the kettlebell with your left hand through the handle in an underhand grip. See Chapter 8 for more details on how to achieve rack position.

3. **Press the kettlebell on your left side up overhead, keeping your right kettlebell down at your side (see Figure 5-8); hold for 30 seconds.**

4. **Re-rack the left kettlebell, and bring it down to your side.**

5. **Bring the kettlebell on your right side into rack position by repeating Step 2 for the right side.**

6. **Press the kettlebell on your right side up overhead, keeping your left kettlebell down at your side; hold for 30 seconds.**

7. **Re-rack the right kettlebell, and bring it down to your side.**

Perform two total reps.

To do the waiter's walk, follow the instructions for the waiter's hold, but instead of standing in place, walk for 30 seconds either forward or in a large circle when each kettlebell is in the waiter's hold position (Steps 3 and 6).

To warm up really quickly with the waiter's walk, switch sides while you're walking instead of standing still as you do so.

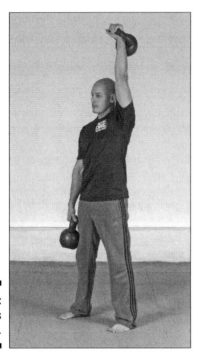

Figure 5-8:
The waiter's hold.

Challenging your joints with Z-Health warm-up options

Z-Health is a mobility program that doesn't use any weight in its exercises. The exercises challenge your joint flexibility and mobility by targeting your nervous system. Incorporating Z-Health warm-up exercises into your routine is one of the best ways to prepare your body for the fast-moving pace of your kettlebell exercises. (Check out www.zhealth.net for more about this program.)

When I incorporate Z-Health exercises in my warm-ups (and sometimes during my rest breaks), I feel stronger and more in tune with my body during my kettlebell workouts. In addition, I recover more quickly and feel much more mobile as a result of Z-Health's very simple movements. To see what I mean, try adding these three simple but powerful movements to your warm-up.

The toe pull

The *toe pull* helps increase your foot mobility. Although you may not think this simple exercise will help your workouts much, trust me: Keeping or increasing your foot mobility goes a long way toward increasing your athletic performance and your everyday movements. So take 30 seconds and add this exercise to your warm-up.

To do the toe pull, make sure you're standing on a soft surface or an elevated booster like a foam roller and follow these steps:

1. **Stand with your spine tall and your shoulders relaxed.**

2. **Using a chair or doorway for balance, put your left leg behind you with the left knee slightly bent and your toes on the floor; curl your toes under your foot (see Figure 5-9).**

   In this position, you should feel a mild stretch on the top of your foot, where the tongue of your shoe usually sits.

3. **Keep your spine tall and look straight ahead as you slowly press or pulse just your toes into the ground; bend your right knee slightly while pulsing to assist you in gently increasing the stretch.**

Perform three to five repetitions on the left side; then switch sides and do the same number of reps on the right side.

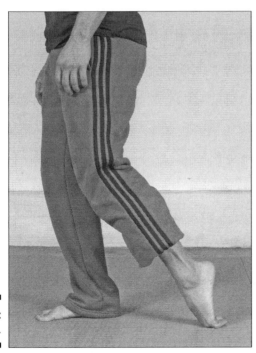

Figure 5-9:
The toe pull.

The knee circle

You've most likely seen or done a variation of the *knee circle* before. Typically, you do this exercise with your hands over your knee caps, but you do the Z-Health knee circle a little differently (which you can see in the steps that follow). The knee circle exercise is great for maintaining and increasing knee mobility and knee health, so it's a great exercise to add to your kettle-bell warm-up.

To do the knee circle, follow these steps:

1. **Stand with your feet about shoulder width apart, spine tall, knees locked, and shoulders relaxed.**

2. **Keeping your feet and ankles relaxed, trace a circle to the right with your knees by letting your knees drop toward the floor to your right (see Figure 5-10).**

Trace five to ten circles to the right; then switch sides and repeat on the left side.

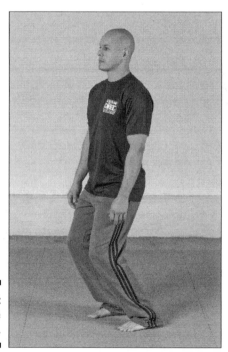

Figure 5-10:
The knee circle.

The shoulder circle

If you experience soreness, tightness, or strain in your shoulders, the Z-Health *shoulder circle* exercise will help alleviate it. Here I illustrate the front and back shoulder circle; you can also do top and bottom circles and circles in a figure-eight pattern.

To do this exercise, follow these steps:

1. **Stand with a tall spine and relaxed shoulders; bring your left arm out in front of you at about hip height with your elbow locked and your hand in a loose fist with your thumb on top.**

2. **Bring your left arm up and out to your left side so that it's perpendicular to your body at shoulder height.**

3. **Trace a circle with your fist by bringing your left arm in toward your body and up above your shoulder (see Figure 5-11a) and then down in front of you to shoulder height (see Figure 5-11b).**

   Concentrate on your shoulder rotating, not your hand, and keep your elbow locked while you perform this movement.

Complete three to five shoulder circles on the left side; then switch sides and do the same number of shoulder circles on the right side.

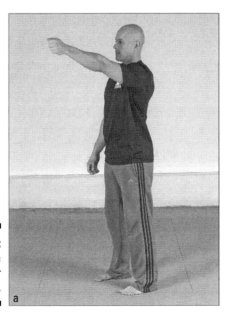 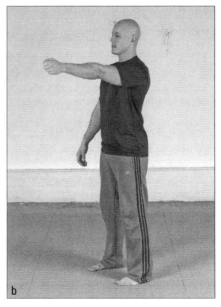

Figure 5-11:
The shoulder circle.

a

b

It's Over! Cooling Down the Right Way

Cooling down your body after your kettlebell routine is just as important as warming it up before, so be sure not to skip your cool-down even if you're short on time. Take at least a few minutes to bring your heart rate down by incorporating two or three of the cool-down options I describe here into your routine. Start by choosing one cool-down option from each category in this section; then, as you progress with your workouts, choose the cool-down options that you like best and that your body responds to the most.

You can also use the Z-Health options I describe earlier in the section "Challenging your joints with Z-Health warm-up options" to cool down. So refer to that section if you prefer to use Z-Health training rather than the cool-down-specific techniques I offer here.

Quick 'n' easy stretches for your whole body

After you finish your kettlebell workout, sometimes the last thing you want to do is take time to stretch. I know after I've had a particularly challenging workout, I just want to collapse in a heap on the floor for a few minutes! But getting your heart rate down and stretching out your body needs to be a regular part of your workout routine. This section gives you some great options for short and quick stretches you can do after you get your heart rate down but before you hit the shower.

Stretching your upper body

This upper-body stretch is one of my favorites because it targets the chest, shoulders, and back and always relieves any tightness or soreness I have in those areas. You need a plyometric box or low table about 20 to 24 inches in height to do this stretch (a coffee table works well).

To do this upper-body stretch, follow these steps:

1. **Kneel about 6 inches in front of the box or table, bring both arms up overhead, and bend at the waist to place them on the box or table; keep your arms straight and about shoulder width apart.**

2. **With your head down, gently sit back so your butt approaches or touches your heels as you keep your arms straight and your hands on the box or table (see Figure 5-12); hold this pose for 20 to 30 seconds.**

Perform one or two reps.

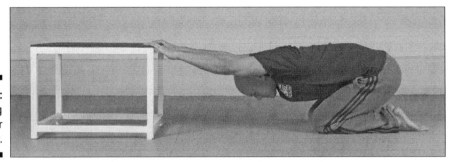

Figure 5-12:
Stretching
your upper
body.

Stretching your lower body

I'm sure you've either done a variation of this lower-body stretch or seen other people doing it. Runners often use this stretch to stretch their hamstring muscles (the muscles in the back of your upper leg). But this variation is more than just lifting your leg and leaning forward to try to stretch your hamstrings. You need a plyometric box or low table about 20 to 24 inches in height to do this stretch (a coffee table works well).

To do this lower-body stretch, follow these steps:

1. **Stand a few inches in front of the box or table and place your left heel on the box.**

2. **With your left leg straight or slightly bent and your foot flexed with toes pointing back toward your head, push back into your right hip as you lean forward to get your fingers as close to your foot as you can, and begin to gently press your foot away from you (see Figure 5-13); hold the pose for 10 to 30 seconds (until you've fully stretched your muscles).**

Perform one or two reps on the left side; then switch sides and repeat the exercise on the right side.

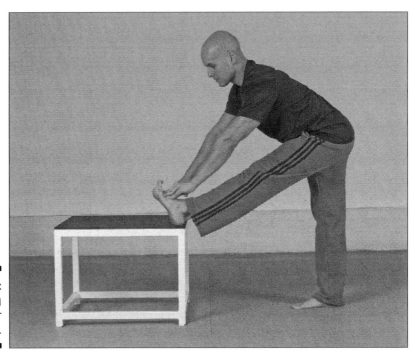

Figure 5-13:
Stretching
your lower
body.

Band stretches for your lower body

If you have a band or strap, you have a couple more options when it comes to stretching the lower body to relieve tired and sore muscles: one for your hamstrings and one for your IT band.

The hamstring stretch

Many people experience tightness in their hamstring muscles. Although the lower-body stretch from the previous section is effective in stretching your hamstrings, I offer you another option here; this stretch requires a band or strap.

To do this hamstring stretch, follow these steps:

1. **Sit on the floor with your legs directly in front of you, and position your band or strap around your left foot above your heel so that you have two parts of the band or strap to assist you in the stretch — one in your left hand and one in your right.**

2. **Slowly lie down on your back as you bring your left leg up (straightened or slightly bent) with your left heel pointing toward the ceiling; keep your right leg straightened on the floor.**

3. **Taking care to keep your hips down, gently pull the strap back toward your head until you feel a good stretch in your left hamstring (see Figure 5-14); hold this pose for 20 to 30 seconds, and then gently release.**

Don't yank your muscles! Always be gentle when pulling back into this stretch.

Perform one rep with the left leg; then switch sides and repeat the exercise with the right leg.

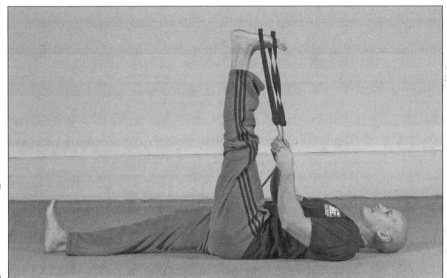

Figure 5-14: Using a band to stretch the hamstrings.

The IT band stretch

Your *iliotibial band* (or *IT band*, for short) is located on the outside of your thigh and runs from the hip all the way down to your outer shin bone. Many people have tight IT bands, although they may not notice them. I offer you a great stretch to help you stretch your IT band here. (Later in this chapter, I show you an IT band stretch using a foam roller, which is especially good if you have a tight IT band and are experiencing knee pain as a result.)

To do the IT band stretch, follow these steps:

1. **Sit on the floor with your legs directly in front of you, and position your band or strap over your left foot so that you have two parts of the band or strap to assist you — one in your left hand and one in your right.**

2. **Slowly lie down on your back as you bend your left leg to a 45-degree angle above you; keep your right leg straightened on the floor.**

   When you bend your left leg, your knee should be above your left side and your foot should be above your midsection or right side.

3. **Take both parts of the strap or band into your right hand, and gently pull it toward your head as you use your left hand to gently press your knee in the opposite direction, taking care to keep the left leg at a 45-degree angle (see Figure 5-15); hold the stretch for 10 to 30 seconds.**

Perform one rep on the left side; then switch sides and repeat the exercise on the right side.

Foam roller release stretches

If you have a foam roller, try using the following three soft-tissue-releasing techniques to stretch your upper- and lower-body after your kettlebell work-out. If you don't have a foam roller, you may want to buy one if you can afford it because the benefits you get from doing these stretches are well worth the price of a roller. (A good foam roller typically costs from $25 to $45, and some rollers come with educational media — DVDs or exercise sheets — that show you how to do a range of stretches for your entire body.)

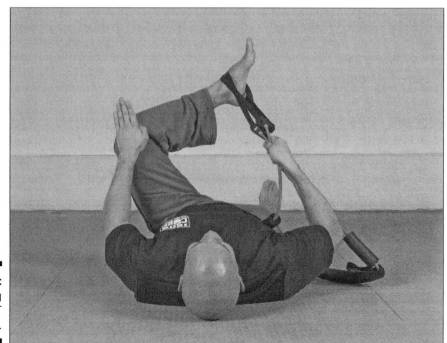

Figure 5-15: Stretching your IT band.

The upper-body foam roller stretch

This upper-body foam roller stretch not only relieves tension and sore muscles but also helps improve spine mobility.

To do this stretch, follow these steps:

1. **Sit on the ground with your foam roller positioned on the floor behind your lower back.**

2. **With your hands behind your back, slowly lie down and roll the foam roller toward your upper back, keeping your back flat (see Figure 5-16).**

   Bend your knees and keep your feet on the ground in front of you to assist you in rolling the foam roller throughout the movement.

3. **Slowly roll the foam roller back and forth between your upper and lower back, taking care to find the areas that have a lot of tension and holding the foam roller beneath those areas until you no longer feel the tension; continue rolling until all tension, soreness, and tightness have been released.**

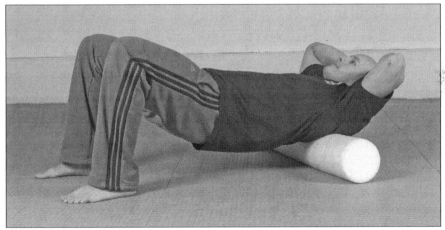

Figure 5-16: The upper-body foam roller stretch.

The hamstring foam roller stretch

People with tight hamstrings have some limitations when it comes to sitting back into their hips during kettlebell exercises. So if you have tight hamstrings, get a foam roller and do the exercise I describe here. A foam roller typically provides more relief than a band or standing hamstring stretch because the roller applies pressure to release the tissue around your muscle.

To do this exercise, follow these steps:

1. **Place the foam roller on the floor and sit on it with your knees bent; put your hands behind you on the ground and your feet in front of you to balance.**

2. **Roll the foam roller along the upper hamstring area in the places you feel tightness and pressure (see Figure 5-17). Continue to roll the foam roller gently from your hamstrings to your knees until all tension, soreness, and tightness have been released.**

Using a foam roller gives you a lot of freedom to find all your pressure points. To get the greatest benefit from the hamstring stretch with the roller, adjust your positioning as needed to make sure you hit all the sore spots.

The IT band foam roller stretch

As I mention in the earlier section "The IT band stretch," a tight IT band can cause knee pain, although you usually don't know your IT band is tight. Even if you don't have any knee pain, though, consider doing this stretch because it feels great after you finish it; plus, it helps relieve tightness and tension caused by your workouts.

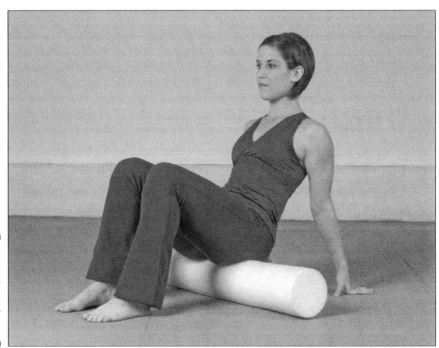

Figure 5-17:
Using a foam roller to stretch your hamstrings.

To do this stretch, follow these steps:

1. **Position yourself on your left side so that your left hip is on the foam roller and your left forearm is on the floor in front of you (see Figure 5-18).**

2. **Roll the foam roller back and forth along the length of your IT band (hip to shin), taking care to find the areas of tension and muscle tightness; continue to roll until all tension, soreness, and tightness have been released.**

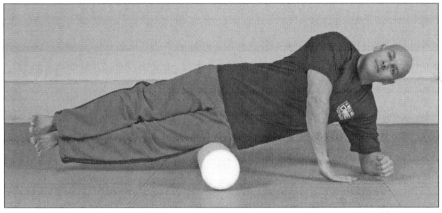

Figure 5-18:
Using a foam roller to stretch your IT band.

Perform one rep on the left side; then switch sides and repeat the exercise on the right side. If you still feel tension or tightness, perform another rep on each side.

Taking Care of Yourself after a Workout

So you've finished your kettlebell workout, but you're not feeling so hot afterward; your muscles really ache! You may wonder how you can tell whether you have serious muscle pain or are just sore. Here's how to distinguish the two:

✔ **Muscle soreness:** Muscle soreness from your kettlebell workout typically begins to set in 24 to 48 hours after your workout. But it subsides when you begin to move around again (by walking, going up and down stairs, and so on). In this section, I provide some solutions for relieving soreness in different parts of your body.

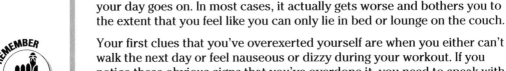

✔ **Muscle pain:** Unlike simple soreness, muscle pain doesn't diminish as your day goes on. In most cases, it actually gets worse and bothers you to the extent that you feel like you can only lie in bed or lounge on the couch.

Your first clues that you've overexerted yourself are when you either can't walk the next day or feel nauseous or dizzy during your workout. If you notice these obvious signs that you've overdone it, you need to speak with your doctor and adjust your workout to meet your current fitness level; I provide some information in this section that can help you do just that.

Surveying soreness solutions

In my experience, new students (even those who are very fit) are sore after using kettlebells for the first few weeks. After the first workout, the areas of soreness are typically the legs and glutes because kettlebells really work those parts of the body. More than one new student has come to me the day after their first workout to say they're having a difficult time going up and down stairs or sitting. Rest assured, as long as you're still able to engage in your everyday life activities, the soreness from your workouts should subside within 24 to 48 hours after you first notice it — just in time for your next kettlebell workout! The following sections offer solutions for relieving soreness in several spots.

If after moving around (partaking in everyday life activities) and doing some of the stretches in this section, you still feel like you can't walk and need to be waited on from the couch, call your doctor because you may have really over-done it during your workout.

Solutions for shoulder soreness

If your shoulders are sore after a kettlebell workout, use the following stretches from earlier in this chapter to help alleviate your muscles:

✔ Downward dog to cobra (see the section "Doing dynamic stretches")

✔ Z-Health shoulder circle (see the section "Challenging your joints with Z-Health warm-up options")

✔ Upper-body stretch from the section "Quick 'n' easy stretches for the whole body"

Solutions for back tightness

If you're experiencing tightness in your back after your kettlebell workout, you most likely need to check your form (especially for the swing, which I discuss in Chapter 6) to make sure you're using your hips to move the weight — and not your back muscles (see Chapter 4 for tips on this concept). In addition, make sure the size kettlebell you're using isn't too heavy. While you try to figure out the source of your back tightness, try the following three stretches from earlier in this chapter to relieve the tightness:

✔ Downward dog to cobra (see the section "Doing dynamic stretches")

✔ Upper-body stretch from the section "Quick 'n' easy stretches for the whole body"

✔ Upper-body foam roller stretch (see the section "Foam roller release stretches")

Solutions for sore thighs and glutes

Most people experience the most soreness from their first few kettlebell workouts in their lower bodies. Because you're trying out a new way to move and use your body, you may tend to squat instead of sitting back into your hips when performing exercises like the swing. Practicing 100 or more squat-like swings can really make your thighs and rear end sore! To help fix the problem, turn to Chapter 4 and practice sitting back into your hips. In the meantime, take a walk or just move around as you would during the day to help relieve some of the lower-body soreness. You can also try out these three solutions for lower-body muscle soreness from earlier in this section:

✔ Body weight squat (see the section "Doing dynamic stretches")

✔ Lower-body stretch from the section "Quick 'n' easy stretches for the whole body"

✔ Foam roller lower-body stretches for the hamstrings and the IT band (see the section "Foam roller release stretches")

If you've really overdone it: Modifying your program for success

If you determine that you've really overdone it during one of your kettlebell workouts, don't quit the program. All you need to do is modify your workout routine to better suit your fitness level. Lucky for you, you can choose from several easy ways to do so. The keys are not to feel like you can't do your workouts without hurting yourself and not to be intimidated because you were so enthusiastic and excited about kettlebells that you did a bit too much the first time. If you follow the guidelines that I provide in this book, especially those related to reps and sets, you should be able to stay with your program even if you overdid it a bit on your first try.

Try to modify your workout using any or all of these suggestions:

✔ Do 50 percent fewer repetitions and sets than what I indicate in this book or what any other workout book suggests.

✔ Use a lighter weight — drop down one size for your kettlebell.

✔ Alternate your workout days so you receive adequate rest.

Chapter 2 offers some suggestions on how to alternate your workout days to allow your body to adequately recover from your workouts. However, if you need to take more time between workouts, feel free to do so. Above all else, listen to your body. Although I don't recommend working out with kettlebells only one time per week, you can spread out your workouts during the week so that your muscles have time to recover. For example, you can work out on Monday, spend Tuesday through Thursday recovering, and then work out again on Friday. After you've done at least two workouts per week for four to six weeks, you should be able to split up your workouts so that you're taking only one or two days of rest in between them. But, at the beginning, it's fine to take more time if you need it.

Going Up a Notch: Adding Active Rest Options to Your Workout

In many of the workouts in this book (specifically, those in Chapters 9 and 13), I offer you some active rest options that add some variety and more challenge to your workouts. Because you probably already know how to do basic exercises like push-ups, I don't illustrate them here. Instead, I focus the following sections on a few exercises that you can use as part of your active rest periods and that you may not be as familiar with: the plank, the jump squat, and the burpee. I provide specific times and number of reps for these exercises in the workouts in Chapters 9 and 13.

Note: The active rest options in this section are best suited for those of you who have fully mastered the basic exercises in Chapters 6 through 8.

For your core: The plank

The *plank* is a fantastic core exercise that also makes for a perfect active rest choice. It strengthens your core, arms, wrists, and shoulders and increases your core stability, which is essential for preventing injury during kettlebell exercises. Holding the plank for more than 30 seconds is a great challenge, but, as you work on it more, you can try to work up to holding it for one-minute intervals.

To do the plank, get in a push-up position with your hands directly below your shoulders, and then position your forearms on the ground in place of your hands (see Figure 5-19). As you hold this pose, keep in mind the following guidelines to get the most benefit from your plank:

✔ Make sure your entire body is level in one straight line (like a plank of wood).

✔ Make sure you squeeze your glutes, thighs, and abs as you hold your body in line.

✔ Don't let your hips sag.

To help you get in the right form, think about pulling your elbows toward your feet. Doing so helps you keep a tight, straight line.

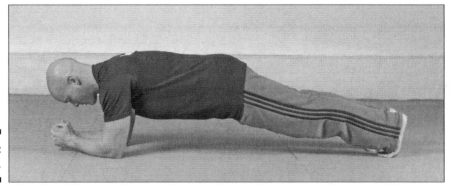

Figure 5-19:
The plank.

For your lower body: The jump squat

If you know how to squat and you don't have knee or other injuries that keep you from jumping, the *jump squat* is an excellent active rest option that keeps your heart rate up and strengthens your lower-body muscles. To do the jump squat, follow these steps:

1. **Get into the squat position with your arms positioned to your sides and behind you and your hands facing up toward the ceiling (see Figure 5-20a).**

   Turn to Chapter 8 for the basics of proper squat form.

2. **In one dynamic, explosive motion, take a vertical leap, bringing your arms overhead to help you up (see Figure 5-20b); then land in the squat position quietly and with soft knees.**

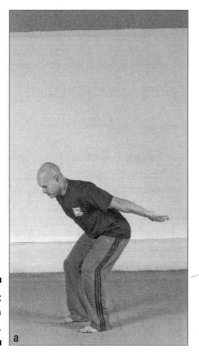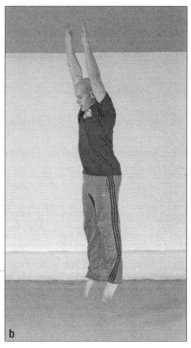

Figure 5-20:
The jump
squat.

a   b

For your whole body: The burpee

The *burpee* is perhaps my favorite active rest option; it's a full-body movement that involves the squat and push-up positions and ends with a jump
squat.

To do the burpee, follow these steps:

1. **Stand with your feet shoulder width apart, spine tall, and abs and
   glutes pinched.**

2. **Squat down with your arms extended and your hands between your
   feet (see Figure 5-21a).**

3. **In one fluid motion, throw your hips back so that you're in the top of
   the push-up position (see Figure 5-21b).**

4. **From the top of the push-up position, perform a push-up.**

5. **In one motion, thrust your hips forward so that you're back in a squat
   position with your arms extended and your hands between your feet.**

6. **From the squat position, perform a jump squat by jumping up into a vertical leap, bringing your arms overhead, and landing with soft knees.**

   See the preceding section for further details on how to do the jump squat.

   If you have knee problems or other injuries that don't allow you to perform a jump squat safely, you can stand up from the burpee instead of jumping up.

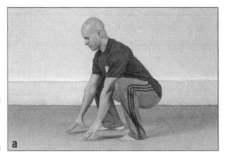 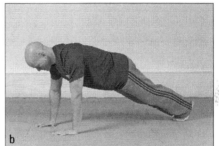

Figure 5-21:
The burpee.

a

b

Part II
Beginning with Basic Kettlebell Moves

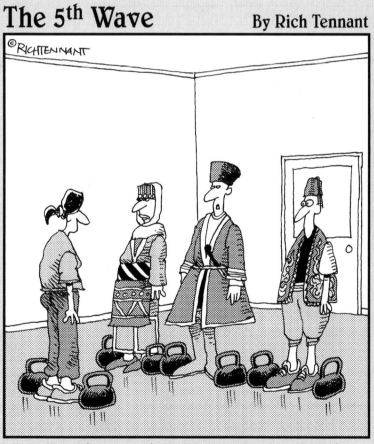

In this part . . .

The basic kettlebell exercises in this part — the swing, the Turkish get-up, the front squat, the clean, and the military press — are your foundation for using kettlebells the right way in all other exercises, so don't skip this part. After you've mastered and practiced the basic exercises I cover here, you'll be ready for some challenging routines. To get started, check out the great programs I include in this part; they can help you see how to put the individual exercises together into a workout and how a typical kettlebell workout should make you feel.

Chapter 6

Swinging Your Way to a Lean and Toned Physique

....

....

You can tell a lot about people by looking at their butts. A strong, firm, and shapely rear indicates that someone knows how to use the glutes and hamstrings for exercise and everyday life, in general. So how do you get a strong, good-looking rear? The answer's easy — lots of swings! The *swing* is hands down the best exercise to make your rear view your best asset. By adding swings to your kettlebell workout, you can achieve incredible gains in hip and core strength while trimming your waist and rear substantially all because the swing is a powerful, dynamic exercise that requires you to control the kettlebell throughout the acceleration and deceleration of the movement. And thanks to the dynamic nature of the exercise, you get a very vigorous cardio workout while using weight, which means you burn tons of fat, too!

So if you're looking for the most bang for your buck, always make swings part of your kettlebell workout. (Did I mention that swinging a big cannonball around your living room is pretty fun, too?) In this chapter, I describe a few practice moves to start with and then describe three effective swing exercises. I also explain some corrective methods in case you have trouble with proper swinging form.

I know you're probably thinking, "You want me to swing that big hunk of iron around my living room? Isn't that a little unsafe?" Don't worry —I explain some important kettlebell safety guidelines in Chapter 2, and, in Chapter 4, I help you discover the essentials of proper hip and spine alignment. Both chapters provide good preparation for you to start swinging. Also keep in mind that mastering the swing ensures success for all the other kettlebell exercises in this book, so perfect this movement before moving on.

Starting in the Right Position and Practicing the Swing Move

Before you conquer the kettlebell swing, you need to get a little practice without the kettlebell first. This nonweighted practice is important because even though the swing is easy to learn, your body likely isn't quite used to moving so dynamically while using weight. Practicing a couple of simple non-weighted exercises before moving on to the kettlebell swing helps you determine whether you're in the right start position, whether you can move your hips properly, and whether you've picked the right size kettlebell — essential basics you need in order to be successful with your kettlebell swing.

In the following sections, you discover the proper start position for swings and practice the swing without the kettlebell; then you move on to practicing the movement by picking up the kettlebell and setting it down, as in a dead lift. After you feel comfortable doing the dead lift, you're ready to perform the two-arm swing and its variations (see the later section "Ready, Set, Swing!" for more information).

Wanting to stop at the top and the bottom of the practice swing is natural, but make sure to keep moving — think of your arms as a pendulum swinging back and forth, and concentrate on driving through your heels as you practice the movement. When you're using a kettlebell, hesitating at any point before finishing your repetitions could cause injury.

Settling into the right start position

When you perform any variation of the swing exercise with or without a kettlebell, you start in the same position. If you're not yet using a kettlebell for this exercise, pretend that you are as you follow these steps to get into the start position:

1. **Stand with your feet shoulder width apart, and put your weight on your heels.**

2. **Rest the kettlebell on the ground between your feet, and line up the handle with your heels.**

3. **Look at a point on the ground 6 feet in front of you, and, as you sit back into your hips, reach down to put two hands comfortably on the kettlebell (see Figure 6-1).**

The proper start position for the swing requires you to push your hips back first and then bend your knees. You aren't squatting down. Instead, think about creasing back at the hips and letting the knees follow. See Chapter 4 for complete details on how to sit back into your hips.

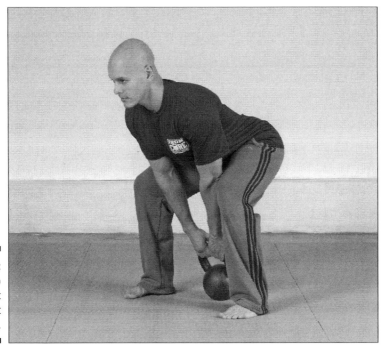

Figure 6-1:
Getting into
the right
start
position.

The practice swing without the kettlebell

Doing some practice swings without the kettlebell is a good way to get your body used to the swing movement. You probably only need to do the non-kettlebell practice swings for a couple of sets before you get the hang of the movement (it's very natural), but you can always perform practice swings between sets if you think your form needs a little tweaking.

To do a practice swing without the kettlebell, follow these steps:

1. **Stand with your feet shoulder width apart, and put your weight on your heels.**

2. **Sit back with your hips, and reach down to put two hands on your imaginary kettlebell (see Figure 6-2a).**

   To sit back with your hips, push your butt back first — like you're trying to tap a piece of glass behind you — and then let your knees bend slightly. See Chapter 4 for complete directions.

3. **Swing the imaginary bell behind you (like you're hiking a football), and aggressively snap your hips forward as you stand up tall; drive through your heels, extend your spine, and squeeze your thighs, glutes, and abs as you bring your arms to chest height (see Figure 6-2b).**

When you perform the "hike" portion of the swing exercise, think about reaching back between your legs, not down. Let your forearms make contact with your inner thighs during this part of the exercise.

4. Without hesitating at the top of the movement, return your arms down to the hike position and sit back into your hips.

Practice ten repetitions so you feel comfortable with the movement.

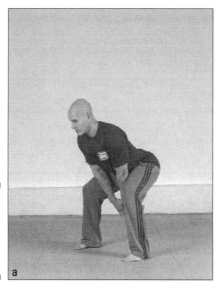
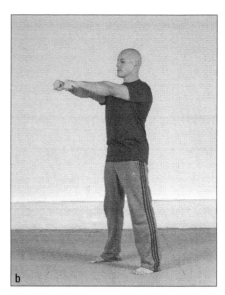

Figure 6-2:
Practicing
the swing
without the
kettlebell.

The practice dead lift with the kettlebell

The *practice dead lift* with your kettlebell is an essential exercise for making sure your body is ready to handle the kettlebell you've chosen to work with. Doing this exercise can help you decide whether you've picked a kettlebell that's too light, too heavy, or just right. (Flip to Chapter 3 for full details on picking the right kettlebell for your needs.) Feel free to do this exercise at the store while shopping for your kettlebell.

In addition, the practice dead lift helps you make sure you're sitting back into your hips properly and driving through your heels while using weight. It also gives you a chance to practice your breathing skills before moving on to the more dynamic two-arm swing, which I describe in the later section "The two-arm swing." (Check out Chapter 5 for an introduction to breathing properly.)

To do the practice dead lift exercise, stand in the start position I describe earlier in the "Settling into the right start position" section, and then follow these steps:

1. **As you pick up the kettlebell, drive through your heels, stand up tall, extend your spine, and squeeze your thighs, glutes, and abs (see Figure 6-3a); your arms are down in front of your body holding the kettlebell throughout the movement.**

2. **As you sit back with your hips, return the kettlebell to the ground, keeping your hands on the bell (see Figure 6-3b).**

   As you sit back with your hips, think about trying to reach back and tap an imaginary wall with your butt. That's the movement you're going for! See Chapter 4 for more information on sitting back with your hips.

   The way you set down the kettlebell is essential to preventing injury. Make sure to complete your rep and finish in your start position, setting the kettlebell down as you sit back into your hips with a neutral spine.

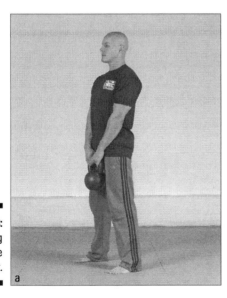 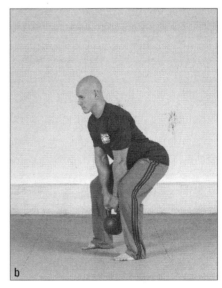

Figure 6-3: Performing the practice dead lift.

a   b

Practice ten repetitions without removing your hands from the kettlebell so you feel comfortable with the movement. Inhale as you push back into your hips, and exhale as you bring the kettlebell off the ground.

While you're bringing the kettlebell off the ground during the practice dead lift and after you've performed ten repetitions, you should feel like the exercise was somewhat of a challenge. If the kettlebell felt like a feather during your practice reps, you need to get a heavier bell before you start practicing swings. Conversely, if you felt a lot of resistance when bringing the bell off the ground and couldn't complete ten repetitions without really working hard, you probably need to get a lighter kettlebell before you start your swings. Opt for a kettlebell size that puts you somewhere in between these two extremes.

In addition to being a great practice exercise before you actually start swinging your kettlebell, the practice dead lift is an excellent glute and hamstring exercise all by itself. After you've mastered the dead lift, keep it as part of your arsenal for getting a strong and great-looking rear.

Ready, Set, Swing!

Are you ready to swing with your kettlebell? In this section, I describe the three basic types of swing exercises. You can perform just one type of swing in your workout routine, or you can mix 'em up and include all three (see Chapter 9 for an effective swing sequence). Whatever you do, keep in mind that performing the basic two-arm swing is more important than working on the variations — the one-arm swing and the alternating swing. As in any exercise program, variety is nice, but you should always include the two-arm swing in your routine.

After you're comfortable with the exercises in this section, perform the following five sets to give yourself a chance to practice your new moves. Try not to rest more than 10 to 20 seconds between each set.

- ✔ **Set 1:** 10 two-arm swings
- ✔ **Set 2:** 10 left-arm swings followed by 10 right-arm swings
- ✔ **Set 3:** 10 alternating swings
- ✔ **Set 4:** 5 left-arm swings followed by 5 right-arm swings
- ✔ **Set 5:** 5 two-arm swings

Of all the people I've taught over the years, I've never met anyone who didn't like to swing. In fact, the swing is usually the favorite kettlebell exercise among students. After all, each set of swings offers a real challenge — and, thus, real benefits. Even if you never increase the size kettlebell you use, you can always increase the number of repetitions you do or try performing timed sets of swings by timing yourself with a stopwatch (rather than counting repetitions).

The two-arm swing

During the *two-arm swing,* you're sure to feel every major muscle in your body working as you swing the bell — especially your glutes, hamstrings, and core. Because the two-arm swing is the foundational exercise for the majority of kettlebell exercises, you need to practice it regularly and to perfection. Over time, the two-arm swing should become a very fluid and natural movement for your body. In addition, you can feel your heart rate increase with each swing, which makes it the ultimate fat-burning exercise.

If you're aggressive in your movement, generate enough force through your hips, and breathe properly, you should experience a big jump in your heart rate from performing two-arm swings. If the movement doesn't seem challenging, consider using a heavier bell.

To do the two-arm swing, stand in the start position I describe earlier in the "Settling into the right start position" section, and then follow these steps:

1. **Swing the kettlebell behind you (like you're hiking a football; see Figure 6-4a) and aggressively snap your hips forward as you stand up tall; drive through your heels, extend your spine, and squeeze your thighs, glutes, and abs as you bring your arms and kettlebell to chest height (see Figure 6-4b).**

   In this top position, your knees are locked out, and your thighs, glutes, and abs are as solid and tight as a column. Forcefully exhale in the top position.

   As you stand up, pretend that someone has your head on a string and is pulling you up. Doing so ensures that your spine is extended and your neck is neutral at the top of the movement.

   Don't use your arms to "lift" the kettlebell during the swing. Use your hips to move the kettlebell. To ensure you're using your hips, make sure the timing of your hip snap is good (see Chapter 4). If you wait too long to snap your hips, you'll use your arms — rather than your hips — to move the kettlebell. As soon as you sit back into the hike position, think "snap hips," and your timing will be perfect.

2. **With complete control, but without trying to slow down the kettlebell with your arms, return the bell back to the hike position by sitting back into your hips.**

   As you sit back into your hips, make sure your weight is in your heels and your spine is neutral (see Chapter 4 for hip and spine essentials).

Do ten repetitions so you're comfortable with the two-arm swing. Don't set down the kettlebell in between reps.

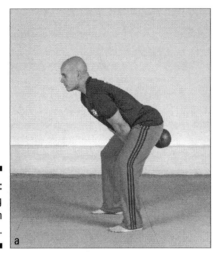 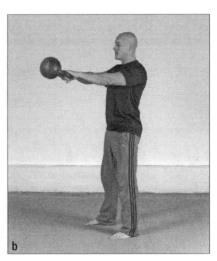

Figure 6-4:
Performing
the two-arm
swing.

The diaphragmatic breathing I discuss in Chapter 5 is especially useful for the two-arm swing because your ability to breathe correctly impacts the amount of force you can generate throughout the movement.

The one-arm swing

After you feel comfortable performing the two-arm swing (see the preceding section), variations like the *one-arm swing* are easy to learn. All the same principles you focus on in the two-arm swing apply to the one-arm swing, except now you have only one hand on the bell instead of two.

Because you're using only one hand to handle the kettlebell, the one-arm swing is more challenging to your body than the two-arm swing. After all, you don't have the benefit of distributing the weight evenly between your left and right sides. As a result, your core has to work overtime to maintain control and stability.

To do the one-arm swing, stand in the start position I describe earlier in the "Settling into the right start position" section, and then follow these steps:

1. **Remove your right hand from the kettlebell and keep your left hand on the bell; your free hand is out to your side (see Figure 6-5a).**

2. **Swing the kettlebell behind you into a hike position with your left arm and aggressively snap your hips forward as you stand up tall; drive through your heels, extend your spine, and squeeze your thighs, glutes, and abs as you bring your left arm and kettlebell to chest height (see Figure 6-5b).**

Forcefully exhale in this top position.

3. **With complete control, but without trying to slow down the kettlebell with your left arm, return the bell back to the hike position by sitting back into your hips (see Figure 6-5c).**

   As you sit back into your hips, make sure your weight is in your heels and your spine is neutral (see Chapter 4 for more on hip and spine alignment).

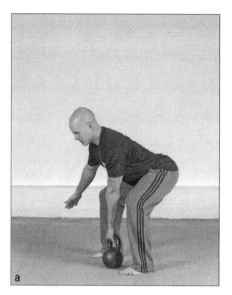
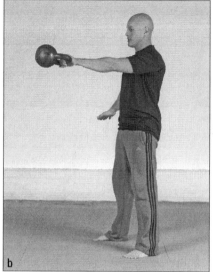
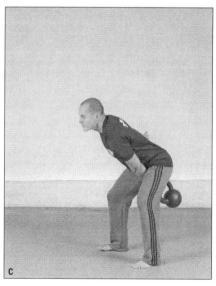

Figure 6-5:
Performing
the one-arm
swing.

Fun facts about the swing

For those of you who are curious about what swings do for you and what size kettlebell you need to use to reap all the benefits, I offer these fun facts:

✔ Your heart rate should be between 160 and 190 while performing 20 swings.

✔ You burn up to 20 calories a minute when performing swings.

✔ To feel the burn even more, you can do the walking swing, which you perform by taking either a forward or lateral step when the kettlebell is at the top of the swing movement.

✔ The average female uses between a 14- and 18-pound kettlebell for swings.

✔ The average male uses between a 26- and 35-pound kettlebell for swings.

Repeat this exercise with the left arm for ten repetitions; don't hesitate at the top or the bottom of each rep, and don't set down the kettlebell in between reps. After you've completed all the repetitions with your left arm, finish in the hike position by sitting back into your hips, and then set down the kettlebell safely. Then do ten repetitions with the right arm.

Don't let your shoulder become disconnected from your lat muscle at any point during the one-arm swing; doing so can cause injury. Control the kettlebell and prevent your shoulder from coming out of the socket by locking your shoulder down into your lat muscle. Refer to Chapter 7 for more details on how to keep your shoulder in its socket.

Rooting yourself to the ground (and not letting yourself come off balance or letting the kettlebell control you) is important for all swing variations, but it's especially crucial during the one-arm swing. To root yourself, forcefully stomp both your feet into the ground before beginning the swing exercise (see Chapter 4 for more details on how to properly root yourself).

The alternating swing

The *alternating swing* is a great exercise for adding variety to your workout, but, more importantly, it teaches you how to properly change the kettlebell to your free hand without having to set it down. For the alternating swing, you're essentially performing the one-arm swing, but, throughout the movement, your free hand shadows your working hand so it's ready to "catch" the bell at the top of the exercise.

You're probably wondering, "Won't I drop the kettlebell if I try to move it from one arm to the other in midair?" Well, you most likely won't drop it if you follow the instructions I present to you in this section, but, just to be safe, you can practice this exercise outside in the yard.

To do the alternating swing, stand in the start position I describe earlier in the "Settling into the right start position" section, and then follow these steps:

1. **Remove your right hand from the kettlebell and keep your left hand on the bell; your free hand is out to your side (see Figure 6-6a).**

2. **Swing the kettlebell behind you into a hike position with your left arm, and aggressively snap your hips forward as you stand up tall; drive through your heels, extend your spine, and squeeze your thighs, glutes, and abs as you bring your left arm and kettlebell to chest height, making sure your right arm is shadowing your left arm as it moves up (see Figure 6-6b).**

3. **At the top position, switch the kettlebell to your right hand, as you forcefully exhale (see Figure 6-6c).**

   Don't let go of the bell until your opposite hand (in this case, your right hand) is on the bell — in other words, for one millisecond, both of your hands are on the kettlebell.

4. **With complete control, but without trying to slow down the kettlebell with your arm, return the bell back to the hike position.**

   As you sit back into your hips, check to make sure your weight is in your heels and your spine is neutral (see Chapter 4 for more information).

Repeat this exercise for ten repetitions, switching sides at the top for each rep. In other words, when you switch from left to right on one rep, you should switch from right to left during the next rep. Be sure not to hesitate at the top or bottom of any rep, and don't set down the kettlebell in between reps. After you've completed all repetitions, finish in the hike position by sitting back into your hips, and then set down the kettlebell safely.

It's easy to lose your timing on the alternating swing and end up switching hands at the bottom in the hike position. This improper form will end up hurting your back, so practice this exercise without the bell first if you're having problems with your timing during the switch.

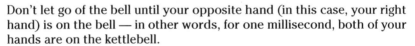

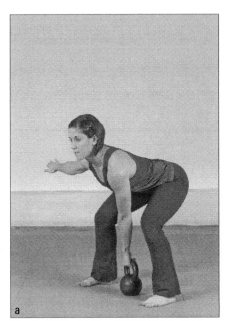
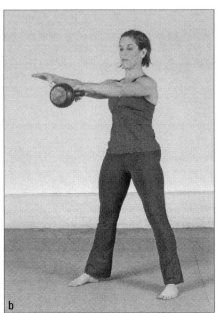
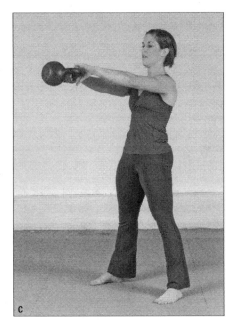

Figure 6-6:
Performing the alternating swing.

Easy Solutions for Bad Swinging Form

To get the most out of your kettlebell exercises, you have to use proper form and technique. But don't worry if you're struggling to maintain the right form; I'm here to put your mind — and form — at ease. New kettlebell students typically make the same mistakes. Based on my experience of working with thousands of students over the years, I've put together a list of form correction techniques to help you get the most from your kettlebell training. Using the corrective strategies in this section will help you quickly pinpoint and solve common swing technique issues.

The dynamic and ballistic nature of kettlebell movements calls for a complete focus on your body and the way it feels while exercising. For this reason, you don't find any mirrors in my gym. But, because you're practicing at home, I recommend using a mirror if your form isn't quite up to par and you think watching yourself exercise may help improve it.

Eliminating back pain with face-the-wall squats

If you have pain in your back while performing the swing, chances are you're not hinging back into your hips properly. The *face-the-wall squat* is a powerful corrective technique that teaches your body to properly hinge back into the hips. Try out this exercise to fix your form by following these steps:

1. **Face a wall with your feet shoulder width apart; stand about 6 to 10 inches from the wall.**

2. **Keep facing forward as you sit back into your hips and simultaneously pull yourself down to about 90 degrees; your arms are at your side (see Figure 6-7).**

   Check out Chapter 4 for a full explanation of how to sit back into your hips.

3. **Drive through your heels, extend your spine as you stand up tall, and tighten your abs and glutes.**

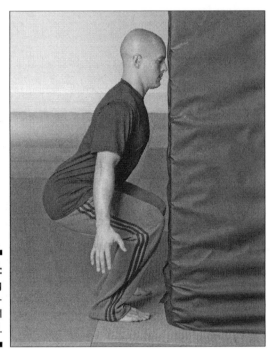

Figure 6-7:
Performing
the face-
the-wall
squat.

Practice ten repetitions of this exercise. Then grab your kettlebell and perform ten two-arm swing repetitions away from the wall, keeping the same hinge in your hips as you sit back to hike the bell behind you. You should notice a difference in your form, and your back should no longer hurt as you swing.

Think hips *then* knees when performing the swing — the hips go back first and the knees follow. Don't get confused; the swing is *not* a squat! The face-the-wall squat is merely a convenient name for this corrective exercise that helps you hinge better at the hips.

Making your hips do the work with the towel swing

People often try to use their arms to "lift" the kettlebell up from between their legs during a swing instead of letting the hips do the work. If you're in the same boat, you may have tight hips, or, more likely in fact, you may just be conditioned to lift weights without engaging your core and hips.

How do you know you're lifting with your arms and not your core and hips? A clear indication is that the bottom of your kettlebell isn't facing forward at the top of the swing. Instead, it's facing downward, and you're basically holding it up with your arms.

The *towel swing* is a perfect solution to this issue because it doesn't allow you to swing the bell with your arms — it forces you to use your hips. For this exercise, you need a small hand-sized towel and your kettlebell. To do the towel swing, follow these steps:

1. **Start in the swing position I describe earlier in the "Settling into the right start position" section, but have your kettlebell face sideways between your feet.**

2. **Place the towel through the kettlebell's handle so you have two "handles" with the towel, and get a tight grip on the towel.**

3. **Pin your elbows into your rib cage, swing the kettlebell behind you, and aggressively snap your hips forward as you stand up tall; drive through your heels, extend your spine, and squeeze your thighs, glutes, and abs as you bring your arms and kettlebell to midstomach height (see Figure 6-8a).**

   Forcefully exhale in the top position.

   Don't let your elbows leave your rib cage. If you do, your kettlebell could get out of control. Instead, keep your arms pinned to your body to ensure control — the idea isn't to swing high but to keep the movement about midstomach height.

4. **With complete control, but without trying to slow down the kettlebell with your arms, return the bell back to the hike position (see Figure 6-8b).**

Practice ten repetitions of this exercise; make sure you don't hesitate at the bottom or the top of the exercise, and don't set down the kettlebell between reps. After you've completed all repetitions, finish in the hike position by sitting back into your hips, and then set down the kettlebell safely. Then take the towel off the handle and perform ten repetitions of the two-arm swing, which I describe in the earlier section "The two-arm swing." After doing the towel swing, you should notice that you're hinging more into the hips.

The towel swing can be a substitute for the two-arm swing for as long as you need it to be. So use this corrective strategy until you've mastered sitting back into your hips.

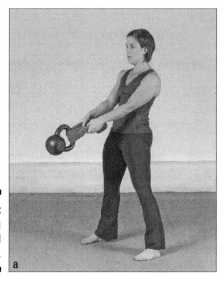 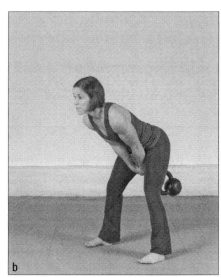

Figure 6-8:
Performing
the towel
swing.

a

b

Think of your arms as ropes and your hands as hooks throughout any of the swing variations. Your hips do all the work; your arms are just the guide.

Combating knee pain with box squats

If you're having pain in your knees while performing the swing, you're most likely squatting down rather than hinging back into the hips. In addition, you may be letting your knees come past your toes. Your weight always needs to be resting in your heels. Try out the face-the-wall squat, which I describe in the "Eliminating back pain with face-the-wall squats" section, to correct your form and technique. If the face-the-wall squat doesn't eliminate the knee pain, try the box squat, which I describe here.

The *box squat* is a great corrective strategy for eliminating knee pain from performing the swing. Take a chair or a small sturdy box with enough surface area for your rear end. A plyometric box works well, but a Reebok stepper or BOSU Balance Trainer also works.

To do the box squat, follow these steps:

1. **Place your chair or box behind you, and take one full step forward.**

2. **Hold your hands out in front of you, put your weight in your heels, and reach back for the chair or box with your hips then rear (see Figure 6-9).**

3. **Tap the box or chair with your rear end, and aggressively drive through your heels and snap your hips as you stand up tall.**

   You may feel like you're going to fall back into the chair, but keeping the weight in your heels helps steady you.

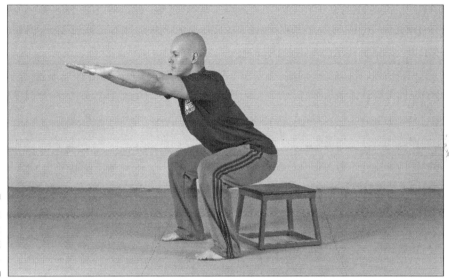

Figure 6-9:
Performing
the box
squat.

Practice ten repetitions of this exercise. Then grab your kettlebell and practice ten two-arm swings. After practicing the box squat and trying another set of swings, you shouldn't feel any knee pain. If you still do, continue to work on this corrective technique and alternate between performing the two-arm swing and practicing the corrective technique. (Flip to Chapter 8 if you're interested in doing box squats with your kettlebell.)

Chapter 7

Turkish Delight: Tackling the Turkish Get-Up

• •

In This Chapter

▶ Working on the Turkish get-up without extra weight

▶ Performing different versions of the Turkish get-up with a kettlebell

▶ Fixing your Turkish get-up form

• •

*O*ver the years, the *Turkish get-up (TGU)* has humbled many seemingly strong and fit new kettlebell students, but, with a bit of practice and concentration, you'll be able to do it well — although I can't promise the TGU will be on your list of favorite kettlebell exercises! Seriously, though, the Turkish get-up isn't as torturous as it sounds. It's a challenging exercise that unmasks your body's weak points by doing the following:

✔ **Working your core muscles:** The TGU teaches all your core muscles (also known as *stabilizer muscles*) — which generally are weak from either not being used or not getting a full workout during your machine-based exercises — how to work together to move your body from lying on the ground to standing, all while holding a kettlebell overhead.

✔ **Strengthening your shoulders:** The positioning of the kettlebell throughout the TGU exercise builds your shoulders' strength, flexibility, and mobility.

✔ **Building stamina in your core and shoulders:** As you work through multiple repetitions of the TGU without setting down the kettlebell, you build an unmatched amount of stamina in your core and shoulders.

As you practice and master the Turkish get-up, your core muscles communicate with your shoulders and lower half to get your whole body to work like one well-orchestrated band, which is an important skill for your body to master because all the muscles of your body move together as one unit in everyday life. For example, all your muscles need to work together for you to get up from a chair, to walk down the street, or simply to pick something up from the floor. Most people don't think of their bodies as consisting of many parts that have to work together, but your kettlebell training surely makes this fact evident — and nowhere is this fact more apparent than with the TGU exercise.

In this chapter, I show you how to practice the TGU without any weight so you can get used to the necessary arm and leg movements. I then describe several variations of the TGU and several strategies to ensure that your form is in tiptop shape.

Don't attempt to do the TGU with your kettlebell until you've mastered the footwork first. Also, keep your eyes on your kettlebell throughout the entire exercise; if you take your eyes off the kettlebell during the movement, you risk breaking your elbow lock, which messes up your form.

Practicing the Turkish Get-Up without a Kettlebell

Practicing the TGU without a kettlebell first is extremely important. The TGU is almost like a dance move in that it requires you to go through the exercise step by step and master each part before moving to the next one. Also, the exercise is challenging enough without weight, and you may encounter problems if you try to use your kettlebell before your body is ready.

In the following sections, I describe how to perform two practice moves: the nonweighted half Turkish get-up and the nonweighted full Turkish get-up. (Later in this chapter, I explain how to perform these exercises with weight.)

If you prefer to hold something as you practice the TGU, you can use a 2-pound dumbbell or a small palm-sized medicine ball of the same weight. Take your time throughout the steps in the following sections and practice the non-kettlebell TGU until you can go through the movements easily.

The nonweighted half Turkish get-up

Performing the *nonweighted half TGU* (the half TGU without a kettlebell) helps you master the first part of the TGU exercise before you move on to the more complicated steps of the full TGU (which I describe in the next section). It also helps you make sure your shoulder and arm are in the proper position before you add weight to the exercise. This exercise can be difficult to master, so take your time and stay focused.

Keep your shoulder fully engaged and connected to the lat muscle throughout this exercise. If you're uncertain what I mean, see the "Maintaining shoulder connection with a simple partner exercise" section later in this chapter.

To do the nonweighted half TGU, follow these steps:

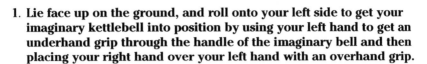

1. **Lie face up on the ground, and roll onto your left side to get your imaginary kettlebell into position by using your left hand to get an underhand grip through the handle of the imaginary bell and then placing your right hand over your left hand with an overhand grip.**

   Keep your eyes on your imaginary kettlebell throughout the movement.

2. **As you roll back onto your back, bring your imaginary bell to your chest with both hands; at the same time, bend your left knee to a 90-degree angle, keeping your left foot and heel on the ground (see Figure 7-1a).**

3. **Press the imaginary kettlebell up with your left hand, using your right hand to assist you; fully lock out your left elbow and release your right hand to the ground so it is positioned on your right side at about 45 degrees with your palm facing down (see Figure 7-1b).**

4. **Pushing your right elbow into the ground, aggressively sit up at a 45-degree angle, keeping the left elbow fully locked out (see Figure 7-1c).**

   Don't try to sit straight up. Keep your working arm (your left arm) stable, and don't move it forward or backward throughout the exercise.

5. **Come to a fully upright, seated position (see Figure 7-1d).**

   Your left knee is still bent at a 90-degree angle with your left heel on the ground, your left elbow is still locked out, and your right arm is still at a 45-degree angle, palm on the ground. Continue to keep your eyes on the imaginary kettlebell.

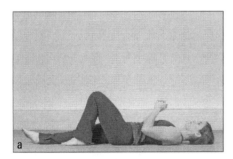
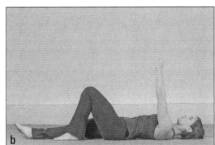
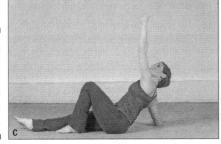
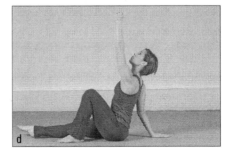

Figure 7-1:
Practicing the non-weighted half Turkish get-up.

6. **From the seated position, slowly and in a controlled motion, lie back down to the start position I describe in Step 2.**

Keeping your arm straightened and your elbow locked, repeat Steps 2 through 6 for five reps on the left side. When you're finished with your reps on the left, use both hands to bring the imaginary kettlebell back to your chest, slowly roll onto your left side, and gently place the imaginary kettlebell on the ground. Then switch sides and do five reps on the right side.

The nonweighted full Turkish get-up

After you've mastered the nonweighted half TGU in the preceding section, you're ready to move to the *nonweighted full TGU*. To do this exercise, follow Steps 1 through 5 from the section "The nonweighted half Turkish get-up" on the left side and then continue with the following steps:

1. **From the seated position, with your left knee still bent at a 90-degree angle, push the heel of your left foot into the ground and the palm of your right hand into the ground to help you lift your hips as you sweep your right leg back and under you (see Figure 7-2a).**

   Your body is in somewhat of a *T* position and your left arm is still fully locked out.

2. **From the *T* position, come to a lunge position with your right knee still on the ground and your left arm pressed overhead in a full lock-out position (see Figure 7-2b).**

   To get into the lunge position, bend your left knee so that your left thigh is parallel to the ground, square your hips with your shoulders, and plant your left heel on the ground.

3. **From the lunge position, stand up tall, pushing through the heel of your left foot, and bring your feet together, taking care to keep the left arm overhead with your elbow fully locked out (see Figure 7-2c).**

4. **From the standing position, reverse the movement; step back into the lunge position I describe in Step 2 by bringing the right knee back to the ground.**

5. **From the lunge position, drop your right hand to the ground to get back into the *T* position I describe in Step 1.**

6. **From the *T* position, sweep your right leg forward so you're back in the seated position.**

7. **In a slow and controlled movement, lie back down, still bending your left knee at a 90-degree angle.**

Practice four reps (Steps 1 through 7 make up one rep) on the left side, and then practice four reps on the right side.

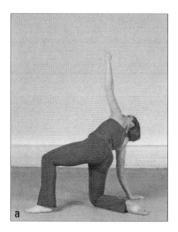 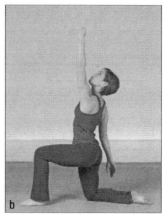

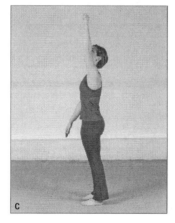

Figure 7-2:
Practicing the non-weighted full Turkish get-up.

Mastering the Turkish Get-Up Progression

The Turkish get-up doesn't require you to do many repetitions to get great benefits. At my gym, Iron Core, students typically use the TGU as a warm-up exercise and perform three to five reps on each side for one to two sets. Sounds easy, right? After you add a challenging-sized kettlebell, this exercise can be brutal, but, within a few weeks, you'll notice upper-body and core-strength gains — which is why it's well worth your time and effort to keep this exercise in your routine at least twice a week.

In the following sections, I explain how to settle into the correct start position for the TGU with a kettlebell and describe four TGU variations: the half TGU, the full TGU, the overhead squat TGU, and the tactical TGU.

The two keys to being successful in any variation of the TGU are

✔ **Sitting up aggressively at a 45-degree angle:** Use your nonworking elbow and hand to help you sit up aggressively. Using your free hand isn't cheating!

✔ **Keeping the working elbow fully locked out:** Keep your shoulder in the socket and your eyes following the bell at all times to help you make sure your working elbow stays locked out throughout the exercise.

Settling into the right start position with a kettlebell

When you perform any variation of the TGU with a kettlebell, you start in the same position. Follow these steps to get into that start position (you can use a yoga mat to soften the ground for this exercise if you want to):

1. **Lie face up on the ground, and roll onto your left side to get your kettlebell into position with both hands by using your left hand to get an underhand grip through the handle of the bell and then placing your right hand over your left hand with an overhand grip (see Figure 7-3a).**

   Keep your eyes on your kettlebell throughout the movement.

2. **As you roll back onto your back, bring the kettlebell to the left side of your chest with both hands; at the same time, bend your left knee to a 90-degree angle, keeping your left foot and heel on the floor (see Figure 7-3b).**

3. **From this position, press the kettlebell up with both hands, fully locking out your left elbow and releasing your right hand to the ground so it's positioned on your right side at about a 45-degree angle with your palm facing down (see Figure 7-3c).**

You can start a set of reps on your left side, go through the reps, and then switch to your right side to do the same.

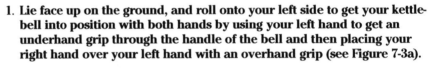

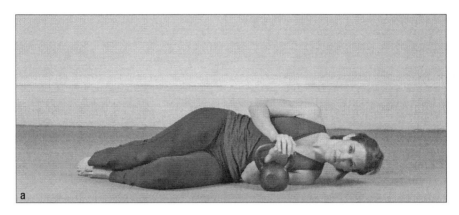

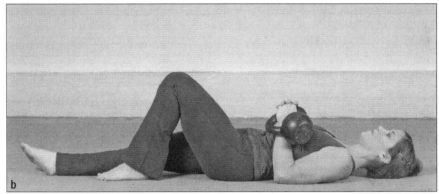

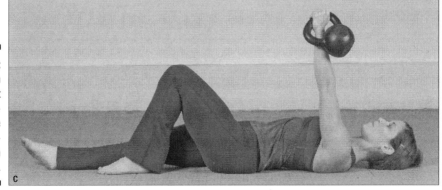

Figure 7-3:
Getting in
the correct
start posi-
tion for the
Turkish get-
up with a
kettlebell.

The half Turkish get-up

It's time to grab your kettlebell and conquer the *half TGU*. To do this exercise, get in the start position I describe in Steps 1 through 3 in the preceding section and then follow these steps:

1. **Using your right elbow to help you, aggressively sit up at a 45-degree angle, keeping the left elbow fully locked out (see Figure 7-4a).**

   Don't try to sit straight up. To help you get up from the lying position while you're holding a kettlebell, shift your weight from your working shoulder blade to the opposite shoulder blade. Doing so ensures that you're sitting up at a 45-degree angle rather than trying to sit straight up.

2. **Come to a fully upright, seated position (see Figure 7-4b).**

   Your left knee is still bent at a 90-degree angle with your left heel on the ground, your left elbow is still locked out, and your right arm is still at a 45-degree angle, palm on the ground. Continue to keep your eyes on your kettlebell.

3. **From the seated position, slowly and in a controlled motion, lie back down to the start position I describe in Step 3 in the "Settling into the right start position with a kettlebell" section.**

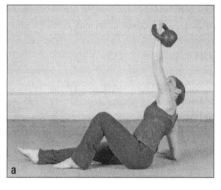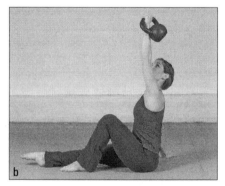

Figure 7-4: Practicing the half Turkish get-up with a kettlebell.

Without bringing the kettlebell back down to your chest (and keeping your left elbow locked), perform four reps on the left side. When you're finished with your reps on the left, use both hands to bring the kettlebell back to your chest, slowly roll onto your left side, and gently place the kettlebell on the ground. Then do four reps on the right side. After you complete all reps on your right side, use both hands to bring the kettlebell back to your chest, roll to your right side, and gently and safely place the kettlebell on the ground.

Never bring the kettlebell over your face or chest to switch it from one side to the other. Set it down, and then either move your body to the other side of the bell or bring it back behind your head.

The full Turkish get-up

After you can perform the half TGU with control and precision, you're ready to move on to the more challenging *full TGU*. To do this exercise, get in the start position I describe in the "Settling into the right start position with a kettlebell" section and then follow these steps:

1. **Using your right elbow to help you, aggressively sit up at a 45-degree angle, keeping the left elbow fully locked out (refer to Figure 7-4a).**

   Don't try to sit straight up.

2. **Come to a fully upright, seated position (refer to Figure 7-4b).**

   Your left knee is still bent at a 90-degree angle with your left heel on the ground, your left elbow is still locked out, and your right arm is still at a 45-degree angle, palm on the ground. Continue to keep your eyes on your kettlebell.

3. **From the seated position, with your left knee still bent at a 90-degree angle, push the heel of your left foot into the ground and the palm of your right hand into the ground to help you lift your hips as you sweep your right leg back and under you (see Figure 7-5a).**

   Your body is in somewhat of a *T* position, and your left arm is still fully locked out.

4. **From the *T* position, come to a lunge position with your right knee still on the ground and your left arm pressed overhead in a full lock-out position (see Figure 7-5b).**

   To get into the lunge position, bend your left knee so that your left thigh is parallel to the ground, square your hips with your shoulders, and plant your left heel on the ground.

5. **From the lunge position, stand up tall, pushing through the heel of your left leg, and bring your feet together, taking care to keep the left arm overhead, the left elbow fully locked out, and the left shoulder in the socket (see Figure 7-5c).**

6. **From the standing position, reverse the movement; step back into the lunge that I describe in Step 4 by bringing the right knee to the ground.**

7. **From the lunge position, drop your right hand to the ground to get back into the *T* position I describe in Step 3.**

8. **From the *T* position, sweep your right leg forward so you're back in the seated position I describe in Step 2.**

9. **In a slow and controlled movement, lie back down, still bending your left knee at a 90-degree angle.**

To complete each repetition of the full TGU, make sure to end in the lying-down position with your working elbow locked out (I describe this position in Step 3 in the "Settling into the right start position with a kettlebell" section).

Perform four reps on the left side. When you're finished with your reps on the left, use both hands to bring the kettlebell back to your chest, slowly roll onto your left side, and gently and safely place the kettlebell on the ground. Then perform four reps on the right side. After you complete all reps on the right side, use two hands to bring your kettlebell to your chest and roll onto your left side to safely place it down.

As with the weighted half TGU, switch sides by passing the kettlebell behind your head (never over it) or by moving your body around the kettlebell.

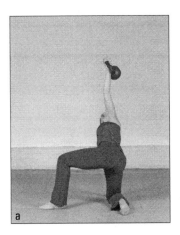
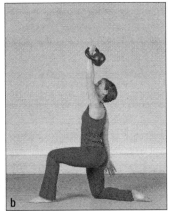

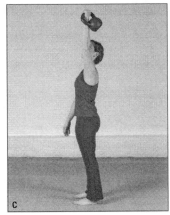

Figure 7-5:
Practicing
the full
Turkish get-
up with a
kettlebell.

If you can do only one good rep on each side, that's fine. Your strength and flexibility will improve to the point at which you can perform three to four reps on each side without putting down the kettlebell between them.

Here are a few ways to make this exercise more challenging (as if you really want to hear them!):

- ✔ Don't set down the kettlebell to the start position until you've completed all your reps for each side.

- ✔ Try out the overhead squat and tactical variations of the TGU. These variations are quite challenging and require a lot of flexibility and control; see the following sections for more details. I don't recommend trying either of these exercises until after you fully master the full TGU and are able to hold your working arm overhead with a locked elbow while keeping your shoulder in its socket.

The overhead squat Turkish get-up

If you can do the *overhead squat Turkish get-up* and do it well, it can challenge you in ways that are different — both physically and mentally — from the full TGU. In addition, the overhead squat itself is an excellent exercise to increase mobility and strength in all your major muscle groups.

The overhead squat TGU requires that you're able to do the full TGU with precision and control and that you possess an exceptional amount of shoulder, back, and hip flexibility and strength. If you're struggling with any part of the full TGU, don't attempt the overhead squat version until you can perform the full TGU with ease. If you can do the full TGU but have trouble with the overhead squat TGU, check out how to fix your form in the later section "Perfecting your overhead squat form"; you also can read Chapter 8 to master the correct rock-bottom squat form and then come back to this exercise.

To do this exercise, get in the start position I describe in the "Settling into the right start position with a kettlebell" section earlier in this chapter and then follow these steps:

1. **Using your right elbow to help you, aggressively sit up at a 45-degree angle, keeping the left elbow fully locked out (refer to Figure 7-4a).**

2. **Come to a fully upright, seated position (refer to Figure 7-4b).**

   Your left knee is still bent at a 90-degree angle with your left heel on the ground, your left elbow is still locked out, and your right arm is still at a 45-degree angle, palm on the ground. Continue to keep your eyes on your kettlebell.

3. **From the seated position, bring your right leg forward and press your right foot and heel into the ground so that you're in a rock-bottom squat position; make sure both heels are on the ground (see Figure 7-6a).**

   See Chapter 8 for details on how to get into rock-bottom squat position.

4. **Using your right hand to help you push up from the floor, drive through both heels and stand up tall, all the while keeping the left elbow locked out, the left shoulder in its socket, and your eye on the kettlebell (see Figure 7-6b).**

   Make sure to keep your weight in your heels and your heels on the ground when you come into and drive up through the squat position. You'll end up off balance and with pain in your knees if your heels come off the ground in this movement.

5. **From the standing position, keep your left elbow locked out, and reverse back down into the rock-bottom squat position I describe in Step 3, using your right hand to guide you down to the ground.**

6. **Slowly and in a controlled motion, return to the seated position I describe in Step 2.**

7. **From the seated position, slowly lie back down to the start position I describe in Step 3 of the "Settling into the right start position with a kettlebell" section.**

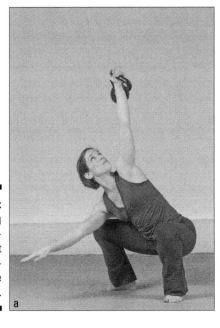
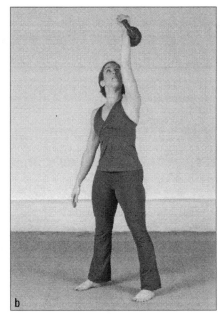

Figure 7-6: Practicing the overhead squat Turkish get-up with the kettlebell.

a

b

Without bringing the kettlebell back down to your chest in between reps (and keeping the working elbow locked), perform four reps on the left side; then set down the kettlebell and either move your body around the kettlebell or pass it around and behind your head to switch sides. Perform four reps on the right side. After you complete all reps, use two hands to bring your kettlebell to your chest and roll onto your side to safely place it down on the ground.

Don't let your knees cave in during the squat portion of this exercise, and try not to twist your torso as you look up at the kettlebell. Doing so will cause knee and back pain. Find corrective techniques for these common errors in the "Perfecting your overhead squat form" section later in this chapter.

The tactical Turkish get-up

Like the overhead squat TGU that I describe in the preceding section, the *tactical TGU* requires a bit more skill and stability than the full TGU. To do this exercise well, you need to be able to lift your hips high off the floor, which requires a lot of core stability and hip flexibility. I recommend that you fully master the regular full TGU before tackling this more advanced version.

Note: I don't often have my students perform this TGU variation, but it's a recent addition to the Russian Kettlebell Challenge (RKC) certification, so if you're aiming to be an instructor, mastering the tactical TGU is a must. See the appendix for more information about RKC instructors.

To do this exercise, get in the start position I describe in the "Settling into the right start position with a kettlebell" section, follow Steps 1 and 2 for the full TGU, which I describe in the section "The full Turkish get-up," and then continue with the following steps:

1. **From the seated position, press the heels of both your feet into the ground so that both legs are out in front of you; pinch your glutes as you raise your hips off the ground toward the ceiling as high as you can without arching your back, keeping the left elbow fully locked out, your eye on the kettlebell, and both shoulders in their sockets throughout the movement (see Figure 7-7a).**

   As you do with the full TGU, use your right arm to help you stabilize your body in this position by keeping it straight and directly under your right shoulder.

2. **With both your legs still out in front of you, sweep your right leg back and under you (see Figure 7-7b).**

   Your body is in somewhat of a *T* position; your left elbow is still fully locked out, your left shoulder is in its socket, and your eyes are on the kettlebell.

3. **From the *T* position, sweep your right leg forward in front of you so that both your legs are out in front of you again; pinch your glutes as you raise your hips off the ground toward the ceiling as high as you can without arching your back, keeping the left elbow fully locked out, your eye on the kettlebell, and both shoulders in their sockets throughout the movement (refer to Figure 7-7a).**

4. **In a slow and controlled movement, lie back down to the start position I describe in Step 3 in the section "Settling into the right start position with a kettlebell."**

To complete each repetition of the tactical TGU, make sure to end in the lying-down position with your working elbow locked out. Practice four reps on the left side. When you're finished with your reps on the left, use both hands to bring the kettlebell back to your chest, slowly roll onto your left side, and gently and safely place the kettlebell on the ground. Switch the kettlebell to your right side either by passing the bell behind your head or by moving your body around the kettlebell. Then do four reps on the right side.

Figure 7-7:
Performing
the tactical
Turkish
get-up.

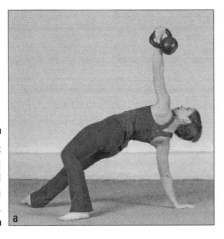
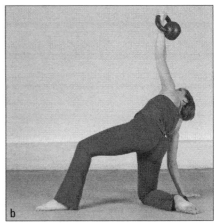

a   b

Correcting Your Form during the Turkish Get-Up

By practicing the TGU again and again, you can gain strength, stamina, and mobility, and by working on the following corrective exercises, you can ensure that your overall TGU form is good, too. The most common form mistakes I run into with new TGU students are (1) not keeping the shoulder engaged in the lat muscle and (2) not keeping the elbow locked throughout the entire exercise. I see a few repeated errors related to the overhead squat form, too, so I address them in this section, as well.

Maintaining shoulder connection with a simple partner exercise

Keeping your shoulder connected to your lat muscle is an important concept for all the kettlebell exercises, but it's especially important for the TGU and swing exercises (see Chapter 6 for more about swings). Most people don't know what it feels like to keep their shoulders in the sockets when performing exercise, which is where this corrective drill comes in.

If you have a shoulder injury, don't perform this corrective drill. See the overhead lockout drill in the next section for more appropriate choices.

To complete this simple drill, you need a partner — ask your spouse or friend to spare a minute to help you. After you have a partner, follow these steps without a kettlebell:

1. **Lie face up on the floor with your legs flat on the floor, and bring one arm up as if you're going to get your arm in position to do the TGU.**

   Make a fist for this drill; don't use a kettlebell.

2. **Have your partner stand over you and wrap his or her two hands around the forearm of your extended arm and very gently pull on your arm (see Figure 7-8a).**

   Notice that your shoulder comes right out of the socket.

3. **Have your partner release your arm.**

4. **From the same position, pull your shoulder back and down into the socket and tighten your abs. Have your partner try again to pull you up using two hands wrapped around your forearm.**

   This time, your partner should be able to pull you a few inches off the ground while your shoulder maintains its position in the socket (see Figure 7-8b). You shouldn't feel any movement or displacement in your shoulder.

   When your partner tries to pull your arm up the second time, he or she may need to apply a little more force, but make sure you're in the right position first; otherwise, you may be setting yourself up for injury.

Practice three reps on each side, and then perform three TGUs on each side, applying the corrective strategy you just practiced. You should feel a difference in how your shoulder sits down in its socket. Throughout each exercise, your shoulder should feel sunk in the socket and connected to your lat muscle. Taking the time to practice this drill a few times and then applying it to the TGU will make a big difference in your overall training.

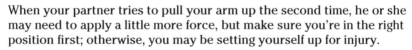

Figure 7-8:
Performing
the partner
exercise for
shoulder
connection.

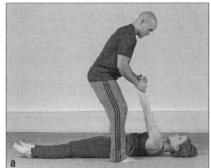
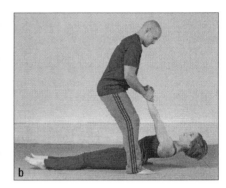

Keeping your shoulder in its socket and your elbow locked

The *overhead lockout drill* is a corrective exercise you can do without a partner; it's a good drill to practice to make sure you know how it feels to have your shoulder sunk down into its socket and to have full lockout in your elbow. You can practice this drill as often as you need to, alternating between practicing it and applying its principles to the TGU.

To do this exercise, follow these steps:

1. **Stand with the kettlebell between your feet, with the handle facing forward, sit back into your hips so you can reach the kettlebell, and use two hands to get the kettlebell into position by using an underhand grip through the handle of the bell with your left hand and placing your right hand over your left with an overhand grip; press through your heels to stand back up (see Figure 7-9a).**

   Refer to Chapter 4 for complete instructions on how to sit back into your hips.

2. **From this position, slowly and in a controlled motion, press the kettlebell overhead with your left arm until your elbow is fully locked out and your ear is in line with your bicep (see Figure 7-9b).**

3. **Sink your shoulder down into its socket.**

   As you do so, you should feel a noticeable difference in how the weight feels relative to your shoulder and lat muscle. In other words, your shoulder should feel sunk in the socket and connected to your lat muscle.

4. **Hold this position for 20 seconds; then slowly bring the kettlebell back down into the start position I describe in Step 1.**

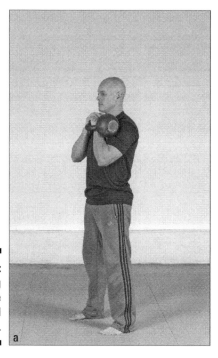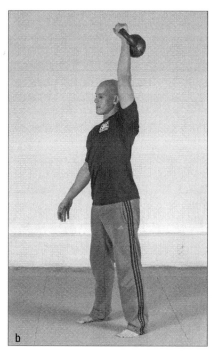

Figure 7-9:
Practicing
the
overhead
lockout drill.

a   b

Practice three reps on each side. Then perform three full TGUs on each side. Like in the partner drill I describe in the preceding section, you should feel a noticeable difference in the way your shoulder feels when practicing the TGU after you do this corrective drill. Your shoulder should feel more sunk down in its socket and connected to your lat muscle.

Perfecting your overhead squat form

Students at my gym who attempt the overhead squat TGU that I describe earlier in this chapter typically make one or both of the following mistakes:

- ✔ Letting the arm fall forward and the elbow break away from its locked-out position while trying to push up from the rock-bottom squat

- ✔ Letting the knees cave inward and twisting the torso toward the arm that's extended while trying to push up from the squat

To build (and maintain) the basic foundation necessary to do the overhead squat TGU well, use a broomstick or other long bar to increase your flexibility and strength. Using the long bar, follow these steps:

1. **Stand with your feet a bit wider than shoulder width apart, and bring your barbell or broomstick up overhead with a wide grip — as wide a grip as you can maintain while still keeping the elbows locked (see Figure 7-10a).**

2. **Perform a rock-bottom squat by sitting back into your hips, keeping your weight in your heels and your spine neutral, and pulling yourself down into a squat; keep your arms wide and pulled back and the elbows locked (see Figure 7-10b).**

   Check out Chapter 8 for full details on the rock-bottom squat.

3. **As you come up from the squat, push through the heels, keeping the elbows locked and arms pulled back, ending up with a tall spine.**

Perform eight to ten reps; then practice the overhead squat TGU for three repetitions on each side. You should feel a noticeable difference in your arm positioning. Doing this corrective drill helps you keep the elbow fully locked out throughout the movement and keep the arm back throughout the movement so it doesn't fall forward.

Focus on pulling your arms back as you perform this exercise — don't let the arms drift forward.

You can also use the band squats I discuss in Chapter 8 to ensure that your knees don't cave in when you perform the overhead squat TGU.

Figure 7-10:
Performing
the
corrective
overhead
squat.

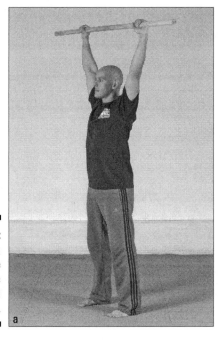

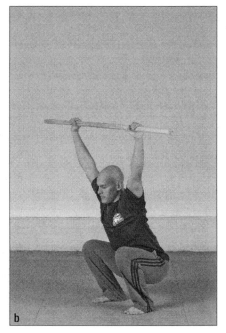

Chapter 8

More Essential Exercises: The Front Squat, the Clean, and the Military Press

This chapter is packed full of three essential kettlebell exercises — the kettlebell front squat, the clean, and the military press. These exercises, along with the swing (see Chapter 6) and the Turkish get-up (see Chapter 7), round out your basic kettlebell routine. With five foundational exercises under your belt, your workout routine will have plenty of variety and challenge for at least the next two to three months (you can find some workout ideas featuring these basic moves in Chapter 9). Indeed, after seven years of exclusively using kettlebells in my workout routine, I almost always include the five basic exercises in my program. And I never get bored of the routine because I've found so many ways to mix up the basics.

To practice the front squat, the clean, and the military press, you use the foundational techniques you learned with the swing and the Turkish get-up. As a result, these three essential kettlebell exercises will be a bit easier to master than the swing and the Turkish get-up. Now that's something to cheer about!

Getting Strong, Sexy Legs, Glutes, and Abs with the Front Squat

Before I started using kettlebells, I was a traditional weight lifter for nearly ten years. Needless to say, I spent many hours in the gym each week trying to get strong but feminine legs and glutes. When I discovered kettlebells, I was amazed at the results I got within the first six weeks of training, especially in my legs and glutes from the kettlebell front squat. And the results came by spending less time in the gym — imagine that!

Your goal for the kettlebell *front squat* is to get into the rock-bottom position (butt touching heels) with good form. What's good form? Think about this: Do you remember when you were a kid playing on the ground or in the sandbox? Children spend a lot of time in the rock-bottom position throughout the day. Unfortunately, with time and age, many people lose that ability. Some of you may have been told by other fitness professionals that squatting past 90 degrees is dangerous. When my clients give me a response like this one when I tell them to get into rock-bottom position, I usually say, "Well, the toilet is past 90, so I know you can do it!" Don't worry if you don't know what I mean by rock-bottom position — the kettlebell front squat shows you how to get there.

The front squat makes it much easier for you to move and prevent injury when doing everyday chores, like gardening, playing with your kids, or picking up heavy things. A couple of added benefits are the strong, nice-looking legs and glutes you'll see thanks to your new exercise. (Do you remember when you had those cute little dimples in your rear end? Well, you can get those back with a combination of front squats and swings — kettlebellers refer to the end result as the "bell butt.")

And don't forget the abs! Although many people don't think of the squat as being a core exercise, if you use proper breathing techniques and good form, the front squat can be a real ab burner. I don't think I've done a single sit-up since I started using kettlebells, and my abs are more defined (except now that I'm pregnant!), leaner, and stronger than I ever thought they could be.

In the following sections, I explain how to get into the correct start position for the front squat and describe how to practice the squat without weight first. Then I show you how to perform the squat with the kettlebell and provide a few techniques to correct issues with your form. (Two of these corrective techniques — the elevated-heel squat and the box squat — are also good options for those of you who are unable to get into rock-bottom position because of major injuries or surgeries. See Chapter 17 for more discussion on using kettlebells as part of your rehab.)

Settling into the right start position for the front squat

When you perform any variation of the front squat, with or without a kettlebell, you start in the same position (see Figure 8-1): Stand with your feet slightly wider than shoulder width apart, your toes pointed slightly out, and your arms down at your sides.

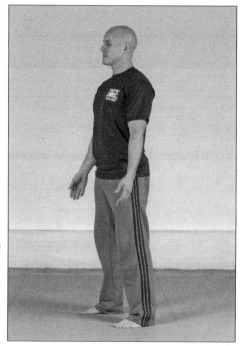

Figure 8-1: The right start position for the front squat.

Practicing the front squat without the kettlebell

To perform a rock-bottom squat safely and with good form, you should practice without the kettlebell first. The following simple exercise can help you assess how good your squat form is right off the bat.

Proper breathing is a must to protect the spine and core during the front squat. Take a deep sniff in through the nose as you descend, and forcefully exhale as you come up, fully engaging your core as you do so. (See Chapter 5 for detailed instructions on breathing properly during kettlebell exercises.)

To do the practice front squat without a kettlebell, begin in the start position I describe in the "Settling into the right start position for the front squat" section and follow these steps:

1. **Bring your arms out in front of you, and, with your weight on your heels, sit back into your hips and let your knees bend as you slowly pull yourself to the ground (see Figure 8-2a).**

   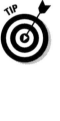

   The goal here is to hit rock bottom (butt touching heels), but if your flexibility and form don't allow you to do so, squat as far down as your current flexibility level and form let you go.

   Keep your spine neutral throughout this movement (see Chapter 4 for more information).

2. **With your weight pushing through your heels and your knees and core stable, drive up to a fully standing position, with your spine tall and glutes pinched (see Figure 8-2b).**

   As you drive up through your heels, be sure to generate force from the ground up and snap your hips to make the squat even more effective (see Chapter 4 for instructions).

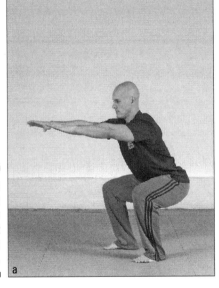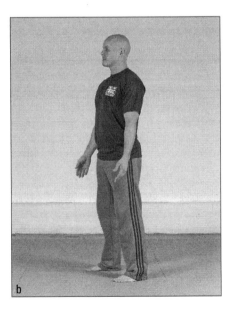

Figure 8-2: The practice squat without the kettlebell.

a   b

Repeat the practice squat without the kettlebell for ten repetitions.

If you were able to get to rock-bottom position without the kettlebell, you're ready to move to the front squat with the kettlebell, which I describe in the next section. If you weren't able to get into rock-bottom position, try the following simple exercise. It's almost always effective in getting new students to a rock-bottom squat without having them go through the corrective techniques I list later in this chapter.

Don't ever use a kettlebell for this exercise because it requires you to breathe through your sticking points (the points at which you get stuck in the squat without being able to go any lower) throughout the squat, and you shouldn't do so while using weight. Continually releasing air from your diaphragm during this exercise puts your core in a vulnerable position and can result in injury if you try to use your kettlebell.

To do this practice exercise, begin in the start position I describe in the "Settling into the right start position for the front squat" section and follow Step 1 of the front squat without the kettlebell exercise (refer to Figure 8-2a); then continue with these steps:

1. **Find your sticking point — the point where you can no longer get any lower — and hold your squat.**

   Keep your spine neutral throughout this movement (see Chapter 4 for more information).

2. **As you hold the squat, take a deep inhale through your nose, and, as you exhale, sink deeper into your squat.**

3. **Continue exhaling through each sticking point until you fully reach your rock-bottom position.**

4. **After you reach your absolute rock-bottom position, with your knees and core stable, drive up through the heels to a fully standing position, with your spine tall and glutes pinched (refer to Figure 8-2b).**

Repeat this practice exercise for five repetitions.

If you can't squat to at least 90 degrees, use the corrective techniques I provide in the "Using corrective techniques for the front squat" section to help you improve your squat form.

You may feel like you're going to fall back on your butt as you approach rock-bottom position. If you do, you can have a partner hold your hands as you go down or use a sturdy door handle for assistance, but don't rely on your partner or the door handle for more than guidance for getting down or coming up. Use your own strength!

Performing the front squat with the kettlebell

Some people who come to my gym don't understand the significance of achieving rock-bottom position in their squats, and, although they could get into position if they really focused, they don't. I recommend you hit rock bottom when you do the front squat with the kettlebell because doing so gives you so much more definition in your legs and glutes and strength in your core than when you go just 90 degrees in your squat. If you still aren't convinced, take note of all the times you squat down to the ground over the next week — wouldn't you rather do so with good form so you can prevent injury?

Your hip flexors are a very important part of the equation for performing safe and effective squats. (In case you're wondering where your hip flexors are, they sit along the crease your body makes when you sit down.) Make sure to engage them throughout the squat. Not sure what engaging your hip flexors feels like? Use this simple partner exercise to help: Lie face up on the floor, and bring your knees to your chest with your legs about shoulder width apart. Place your fingers on your hip flexors. Have your partner wrap her fingertips around your feet, and, as she tries to pull your legs to a straight position, resist the pull using your hip flexor muscles. You want to feel your hip flexors this engaged while squatting.

To do the front squat with a kettlebell, get in the start position I describe in the "Settling into the right start position for the front squat" section; then follow these steps:

1. **Pick up your kettlebell with two hands using both sides of the handle and return to the start position, fully standing and holding the kettlebell close to the body at about chest height (see Figure 8-3a).**

   Holding the kettlebell on both sides with two hands is called *holding the bell by the horns.*

2. **Sit back into your hips as you let your knees bend, keeping your spine neutral throughout the movement, and descend slowly by pulling yourself to the ground (see Figure 8-3b).**

   Aim for getting your butt to make contact with the back of your heels in the bottom position of the rock-bottom squat. Keep the kettlebell in front of you, close to your body, and at chest height throughout the movement.

3. **Without pausing in the rock-bottom position, drive up through your heels, keeping your knees and core stable, to the fully standing position that I describe in Step 1; make sure your spine is tall, and pinch your glutes at the top of the movement.**

Repeat the front squat for ten repetitions.

You should get a vigorous cardio workout when you do rock-bottom front squats. If you aren't out of breath after ten reps, make sure the kettlebell size you're using is challenging enough. (See Chapter 3 for full details on picking the correct kettlebell size.)

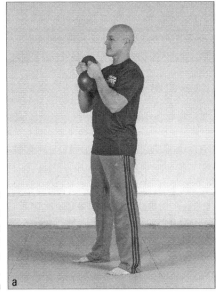 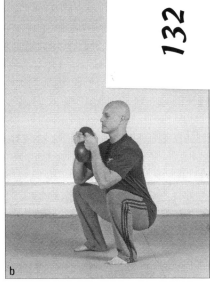

Figure 8-3:
The front squat with the kettlebell.

a

b

If you can get to rock-bottom position with good form, "rack" the kettlebell (see the later section "The rack position" for instructions), and perform ten repetitions on each side. Your core has to work a lot harder to stabilize your body while squatting when you aren't holding the kettlebell by the horns (because the weight is no longer distributed evenly). Also, try doing the *double front squat* by using two kettlebells of the same size in the rack position (left and right) for even more of a core, leg, and glute challenge.

Using corrective techniques for the front squat

From my experience in working with thousands of students over the years, I've found that many beginners make the same five mistakes when trying to perform the front squat:

- Their heels come off the ground as they approach the rock-bottom position.
- Their knees cave inward as they approach the rock-bottom position.
- Their torsos fall forward as they approach the rock-bottom position.
- They descend way too fast, pause at the bottom, and struggle to come back up.
- Their backs round in the descent or ascent of the movement.

Generally, these common mistakes are caused by a lack of flexibility and lack of strength or by an infrequent taxing of your major muscle groups. You can overcome any or all of these form issues by going through the following corrective methods before returning to the front squat with the kettlebell.

Fixing tight muscle problems with the elevated-heel squat

I typically use the *elevated-heel squat* for clients who really lack flexibility and who can't keep their heels down while squatting. It's a simple exercise that gets you to keep your heels on the ground. You may need to use this method of squats for a week or so, alternating between it and the regular kettlebell front squat. If you're extremely inflexible, you may need to use only the elevated-heel squat until you gain flexibility and strength. You can use either a kettlebell or just your body weight to do this exercise.

To do the elevated-heel squat, fold a large bath or beach towel lengthwise to make three or four sections piled on top of one another. Get in the start position I describe earlier in the "Settling into the right start position for the front squat" section, but position your heels on the towel with the rest of your feet positioned on the floor (see Figure 8-4). Then follow the steps for the kettlebell front squat that I describe in the "Performing the front squat with the kettlebell" section.

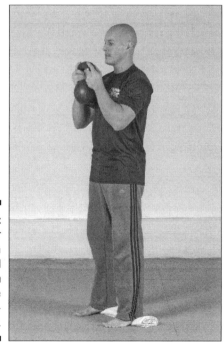

Figure 8-4:
Put your heels on a folded towel to perform the elevated-heel squat.

Repeat this exercise for ten repetitions; then put the towel aside and repeat the front squat with the kettlebell for ten repetitions. You should notice a big difference in your squat after practicing the elevated-heel squat because this corrective technique helps you get noticeably lower while keeping your heels on the ground (or towel).

If you're still having trouble getting into a rock-bottom front squat because of tight muscles, continue practicing the elevated-heel squat, slowly "peeling" layers of your towel away with every few workout sessions until your heels are no longer elevated.

Steadying wobbly knees with the band squat

The *band squat* is one of my favorite corrective techniques (I use this strategy for about 40 to 50 percent of my clients), but it requires a type of band that you may not have lying around the house. You can find one easily at most sporting goods stores and on many fitness-related Web sites, and I highly recommend taking the time to get one if your knee or knees cave inward, if you have a tendency to wobble in any way, or if you experience knee pain while doing the squat. Correcting your form now will go a long way for your knee health and will help you get the most out of your kettlebell training routine.

Note: For this corrective exercise, use a band that's short and tight enough that when you step into it and bring your feet shoulder width apart, it's taut with resistance.

To do the band squat, follow these steps:

1. **Take the band and step into it, positioning it right under both your knees.**

2. **Get into the start position I describe in the "Settling into the right start position for the front squat" section (see Figure 8-5a).**

3. **Proceed with the kettlebell front squat that I describe in the "Performing the front squat with the kettlebell" section; as you squat, push out on the band using your hip flexor muscles, fully engaging your core, legs, and glutes as you do so (see Figure 8-5b).**

   Keep the band right below your kneecaps throughout the movement.

Repeat the band squat for ten repetitions; then remove the band and perform ten kettlebell front squats. If you don't notice a difference in your squat form right away, keep alternating between the band squats and the kettlebell front squat until you're no longer wobbling in the bottom of the squat or letting your knee or knees cave inward during the squat.

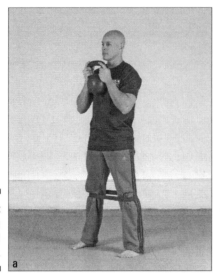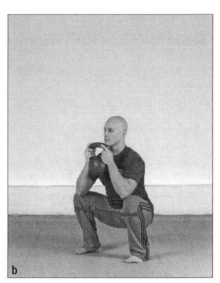

Figure 8-5:
Performing
the band
squat.

The Russian Kettlebell Challenge (RKC) certification course uses a great partner exercise to help students envision "putting space between their hips." While one partner performs the squat, the other partner takes her two index fingers and places them on the squatter's thigh. The partner then drags one finger toward the squatter's hip and the other toward the squatter's knee. This simple cue helps students visualize lengthening from the hip and pushing out through the ground to help them understand how to put space in their hips to get to the rock-bottom position without letting their knees cave inward. If you have a partner, have her try this technique on you and see if it makes a difference in your squat form. You can also have your partner run one finger up your spine toward your neck and the other down your spine toward your tailbone while you're in rock-bottom position; doing so helps remind you to keep your spine tall throughout the exercise.

Getting to rock bottom with the box squat

The *box squat* is a corrective strategy for helping you get into rock-bottom position while keeping your overall form in check. For the box squat, you need a small sturdy box with enough surface area for your rear end — a 12- to 20-inch box or surface makes this corrective technique most effective. You don't use your kettlebell for this exercise. You can alternate between the box squat and the kettlebell front squat until you're able to get to rock bottom without using the box.

To do the box squat, follow these steps:

1. **Place your box on the floor behind you, and take one full step forward.**

2. **Get in the start position I describe earlier in the "Settling into the right start position for the front squat" section.**

3. **Follow Steps 1 and 2 for the kettlebell front squat, which I describe in the "Performing the front squat with the kettlebell" section earlier in this chapter, but don't use a kettlebell; reach back for the box with your hips and rear end as you descend (see Figure 8-6).**

   If you feel like you're going to fall back onto the box, make sure you're keeping the weight in your heels; doing so helps steady you.

4. **Keeping your spine neutral, tap the box with your rear end and drive through your heels, keeping your knees and core stable and pinching your glutes as you stand up to a fully standing position, ending up with a tall spine.**

Practice ten repetitions of this exercise. Then practice ten rock-bottom front squats. After practicing the box squat and trying another set of rock-bottom squats, you should be able to get to rock bottom or close to it with good form.

If you still have problems getting to rock bottom with good form, continue to use the box. It acts as a really good guide and, as long as you have a good sturdy box that's the right height, you can continue practicing your squats this way. A BOSU (see Chapter 3) also works well; just make sure not to "bounce" off the BOSU at the bottom of the squat.

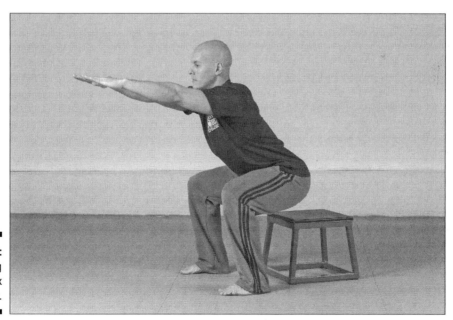

Figure 8-6:
Performing the box squat.

Bringing the Bell to the Rack: The Clean

The *clean,* which is based on the Olympic weight-lifting version with a barbell, is a fantastic exercise in and of itself, but it's also an essential part of getting the kettlebell into the proper position for many other kettlebell exercises. You absolutely need to know how to clean to use kettlebells — so don't skip over this exercise! You can master the clean with the help of the techniques in the following sections.

Settling into the right start position for the clean

When you perform any variation of the clean with the kettlebell, you start in the same position: Stand with your feet shoulder width apart, your toes pointed forward, your arms down at your sides, and your kettlebell on the ground between your heels with the handle facing forward (see Figure 8-7).

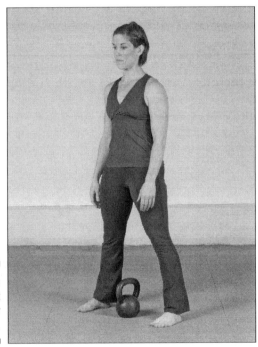

Figure 8-7:
The start position for the clean.

Moving through the clean progression

The following sections offer you a progression through the variations of the kettlebell clean, from easiest to most difficult. I teach this progression to my first-time students in an effort to avoid the most common errors in form. However, if your form needs "cleaning" up after you move through the variations I go over in these sections, check out the corrective strategy I describe in the "Solving form problems with the face-the-wall clean" section.

Before you can move into the clean, you need to get your kettlebell in the correct rack position. After you're comfortable in the rack, you're ready to move on to the beginner clean, the clean, and, finally, the alternating clean. To help you put everything together, I provide a sequence of clean moves that you can add to your overall workout at the end of this section.

The rack position

Getting the kettlebell in the *rack position* is an important step before moving on to the clean with the kettlebell. Before I show first-time students how to do the actual clean exercise, I always have them get in the rack position because, if you don't know how the correct rack position feels, you'll end up racking the kettlebell way too far out to your side or slamming yourself with the bell when you first clean the bell.

To get in the rack position, begin in the start position I describe in the "Settling into the right start position for the clean" section; then proceed with the following steps:

1. **Sit back into your hips and place your left hand through the handle of the kettlebell with an underhand grip; then place your right hand over your left hand with an overhand grip (see Figure 8-8a).**

   Check out Chapter 4 for more details on how to sit back into your hips.

2. **As you stand up, use both hands to bring the kettlebell snug up to your chest with the thumb of your left hand touching your collarbone (see Figure 8-8b); pull your left elbow into your rib cage and release your right hand to your side.**

   Picture yourself hugging a purse strap or backpack strap to your chest; you want the kettlebell to be close to your body. Keep your elbow pinned into your rib cage when you're in the rack position.

3. **Hold the rack position on your left side for 30 seconds; then use your right hand to help you return the kettlebell to the ground by returning it to an overhand grip the same way you started the exercise.**

4. **Switch sides so you get into the rack position on your right side, and repeat the hold for 30 seconds.**

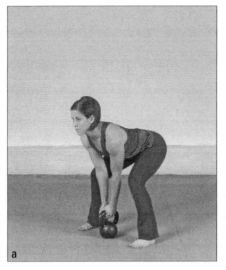
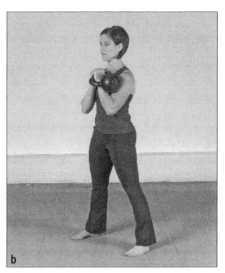

Figure 8-8:
Getting into
the kettle-
bell rack
position.

Complete three repetitions of rack holds (one rack hold on each side equals one rep).

For those of you with large chests or for those of you who feel uncomfortable with the kettlebell on your chest, you can have the elbow slightly away from the rib cage and your kettlebell racked slightly to the side.

Not everyone can achieve a perfect rack position (especially if you have big lat muscles), but no matter what, be sure to keep your shoulder in its socket and sunk into the lat muscle during the entire exercise so you don't risk injury (see Chapter 7 for more on keeping your shoulder in its socket).

The beginner clean

After you know how to get the kettlebell into the rack position, you're ready to progress to the *beginner clean*. The clean is an aggressive movement just like the swing in Chapter 6, but, unlike the swing, this exercise requires you to keep the kettlebell close to your body. The clean really unmasks whether or not you know how to use your hips to move the kettlebell, and, just like in the swing, the timing of your hip snap is essential for good form (see Chapter 4). And, of course, you need to engage your core throughout the exercise, too.

To do this exercise, get in the start position I describe in the "Settling into the right start position for the clean" section; then proceed with the following steps:

1. **Sit back into your hips and reach down and back with your left arm to put your left hand on the kettlebell, taking care to keep your left arm close to your body; rotate your hand inward toward your bell so that your thumb is pointing backward, moving the kettlebell handle to face sideways as you do (see Figure 8-9a); keep your right arm at your side.**

2. **As you bring the kettlebell up from the ground, drive through your heels and snap your hips to clean the kettlebell into the rack position on the left side, ending up with a tall spine (see Figure 8-9b).**

   As you bring the kettlebell off the ground, your thumb goes from pointing backward at the bottom position of the exercise to touching your collarbone at the top of the exercise. Pinch your glutes at the top of the movement, and keep your chest and shoulders square — don't let the kettlebell knock you back.

   Your hips are doing all the work in this exercise; your arm is only a guide.

3. **To return the kettlebell to the ground, sit back into your hips, keeping the left arm close to the body, making sure to rotate the thumb back as you return the kettlebell to the ground between your heels.**

   Don't use your right hand to assist you in returning the kettlebell to the ground. Your right hand stays out to your side during the exercise.

   If you keep your elbow close enough to your body when cleaning the kettlebell, the bell will roll around your wrist at the top of the movement and roll off your wrist as you return the bell to the ground. At no time, however, should it flip or flop on or off your wrist.

Repeat the beginner clean for five repetitions on your left side; then switch sides and perform five repetitions on the right side.

Figure 8-9:
The beginner kettlebell clean.

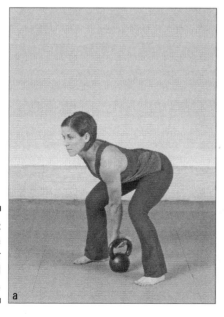
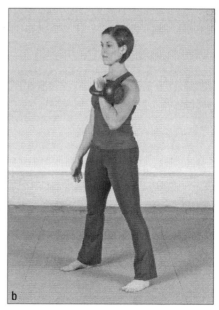

a b

One reason why I have you begin each rep with the kettlebell back by your heels is to ensure that you're at least sitting back into your hips to begin the exercise. Many times when I teach this exercise to new students, they walk backward so the kettlebell handle is closer to their toes! If you notice yourself doing something similar, make sure to reposition yourself accordingly.

I recommend practicing the beginner version of the clean for a week or two before moving on to the clean in the next section.

Think about zipping and unzipping your jacket when performing the clean. Your working arm should stay very close to your body.

The clean

After you master the beginner clean, it's time to move to the actual *clean.* The clean is a powerful exercise for building core, leg, and glute strength. It also works your chest, arms, and back and builds endurance. If you feel comfortable with your beginner clean form, you should be able to move through these instructions rather quickly.

The only difference between the actual clean and the beginner clean is that you don't set down the kettlebell between repetitions. I know it sounds simple enough, but some students run into trouble when they stop putting the weight down between reps. Because you don't set down the kettlebell in between reps, the tendency may be to have too large of an "arc" during the descent and when racking the kettlebell. If you end up smacking yourself, either on the wrist or the chest, check out the face-the-wall exercise I describe later in the "Solving form problems with the face-the-wall clean" section, and practice it until you've smoothed out your clean. The clean (or any kettlebell exercise, for that matter) shouldn't hurt!

To do the clean, begin in the start position I describe in the "Settling into the right start position for the clean" section, and proceed with Steps 1 and 2 from the beginner clean exercise in the section "The beginner clean"; then continue with the following steps:

1. **Keep your left elbow close to the rib cage and rotate your left hand inward so your thumb is pointing backward; as you sit back into your hips, swing the kettlebell back behind you (close to the groin) so that your forearm has contact with your inner thigh (see Figure 8-10).**

   Your right hand is out to the side during the exercise.

2. **Without hesitating in the bottom of the clean position, aggressively snap your hips to clean the kettlebell back into the rack position, keeping your left arm close to the body so that you don't have too big of an arc and end up banging yourself with the bell (refer to Figure 8-9b).**

   The clean isn't a swing, although you do use a "backswing" as you bring the kettlebell out of the hike-like position; keeping the arm close to the body ensures that you don't bang yourself in the chest or wrist.

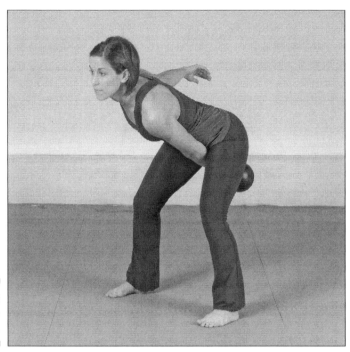

Figure 8-10:
The kettle-
bell clean.

Perform five repetitions on your left side; then either set down the kettlebell or use a swing to switch the kettlebell to the right side (refer to the alternating swing in Chapter 6). Practice five reps on the right side.

The alternating clean

You can perform the *alternating clean* to add more variety to your program or to handle a heavier bell — in the alternating clean, you're essentially performing only one repetition before switching sides. To do the alternating clean, you must have already mastered the alternating swing (see Chapter 6) and the clean (see the preceding section).

Typically, I have my students use this exercise when they're moving up from one size kettlebell to another. But it's just as fun to do with your current size kettlebell, and, because you take a swing in between each rep to switch sides, you get a cardio blast, as well.

To do the alternating clean, begin in the start position I describe in the "Settling into the right start position for the clean" section; then follow these steps:

1. **Complete one clean repetition (Steps 1 and 2 in the section "The clean") on the left side, and, as you're returning to the bottom of the clean position, take an extra swing to switch the kettlebell to the right side (see Figure 8-11).**

   Use the alternating swing technique I describe in Chapter 6 to switch sides safely.

2. **Complete one clean repetition on the right side, and repeat the extra swing to switch back to the left side.**

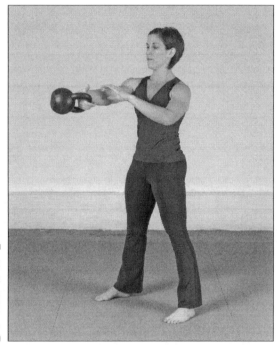

Figure 8-11:
The
alternating
kettlebell
clean.

Perform ten total repetitions alternating between your left and right sides.

Good ol' clean fun: Putting together a clean sequence

Here's a fun and challenging clean sequence to practice the variations of the clean in the preceding three sections. During this sequence, try not to rest between each set, but, if you do need to rest, limit your break to 10 or 20 seconds.

✔ **Set 1:** 10 beginner cleans (5 left and 5 right)

✔ **Set 2:** 5 cleans on the left and 5 cleans on the right

✔ **Set 3:** 10 alternating cleans

✔ **Set 4:** 10 squat/clean combinations (5 left and 5 right)

For the squat/clean combo, clean the kettlebell as in Figure 8-12a; then perform a front squat with the kettlebell in the rack position as in Figure 8-12b. Re-clean the bell before each squat, and continue for five repetitions on each side.

Figure 8-12:
The kettlebell squat/clean combination.

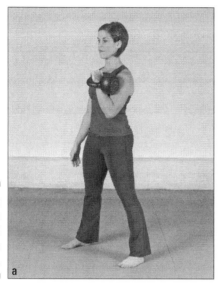
a

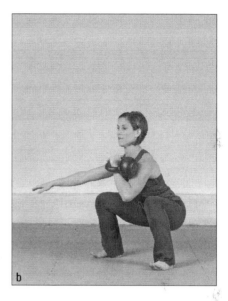
b

To amp up your cleans, use two kettlebells of the same size rather than one. Using two bells is called the *double clean* or simply the *two-kettlebell clean.* You can also have fun with two-kettlebell alternating cleans, but it takes quite a bit of coordination and experience to do that variation correctly.

Solving form problems with the face-the-wall clean

If you notice that you bang either your wrist or your chest as you rack the kettlebell, you probably have too large of an arc when cleaning it. In addition, if you feel the clean more in your biceps than in your glutes, legs, and abs, chances are you're curling the kettlebell rather than cleaning it. Whether you're using too large an arc or are curling the bell, I find the *face-the-wall clean* to be one of the easiest ways to fix most clean problems, and you need to perform only a few reps on each side before you return to the beginner clean or move on to the clean.

To do this corrective technique, you need to have an uncluttered wall space that can withstand a kettlebell possibly hitting it. Even though I can't remember a student ever hitting the wall when doing the face-the-wall clean, it could happen!

To do the face-the-wall clean, follow these steps:

1. **Face the wall and position yourself about 6 to 8 inches from the wall; your feet should be shoulder width apart, and your kettlebell should be on the ground between your feet (see Figure 8-13a).**

2. **Keeping your eyes on the wall, clean the kettlebell as I describe in Steps 1 through 3 for the beginner clean in the section "The beginner clean" (see Figure 8-13b).**

If you're close enough to the wall (granted you don't end up hitting the wall), the face-the-wall clean should ensure that

✔ You keep the kettlebell close enough to your body so you don't bang your wrist when racking the bell.

✔ You keep the kettlebell close enough to your body so you don't bang your chest or knock your working shoulder backward when racking the kettlebell.

✔ You sit back into your hips and use your hip snap to clean the kettlebell instead of curling it.

Practice the face-the-wall clean as often as needed. It's best to alternate between a set of face-the-wall cleans and a set of regular cleans. When doing your regular cleans, keep the visualization of the wall in your mind. Pretending there's a wall in front of you helps keep your technique up to par.

Figure 8-13:
Practicing the face-the-wall clean.

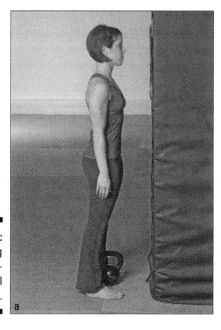
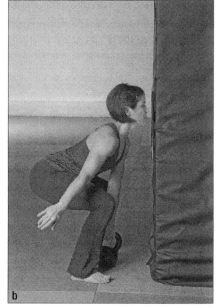

Strengthening and Sculpting Your Arms with the Military Press

One of the biggest appeals of using kettlebells is that the majority of exercises — especially the foundation exercises in this chapter, along with those in Chapters 6 and 7 — work all your major muscle groups. If you did only swings, Turkish get-ups, front squats, and cleans, you'd have a pretty complete program. That being said, you should round out the foundational exercises with the military press.

After you know how to clean and rack your kettlebell, the military press is quite straightforward. If you're a traditional weight lifter, you've probably done lots of presses, but the kettlebell *military press* is different in a few key ways:

- ✔ You fully lock out your elbow at the top of the movement.
- ✔ You fully engage your lat muscles while pressing.
- ✔ You use your core muscles.

The military press strengthens and defines your arms, but your waist gets a nice V-shape, as well. Usually when you work on getting more definition in your shoulders and lats, your waist automatically appears smaller. But the kettlebell military press really engages your core muscles, and using the press along with the clean makes for a fat-burning and ab-, shoulder-, and butt-defining combination (see the "Bringing the Bell to the Rack: The Clean" section earlier in this chapter). I can't remember a workout of mine that didn't include some variation of the military press. Although you don't have to include the press in every one of your workouts, make sure you at least put the exercise in one of your weekly routines.

In the following sections, I describe the basic military press and a couple of fun variations, and I provide pointers on how to fix bad press form.

Doing the basic military press

To do the military press, follow these steps:

1. **Rack your kettlebell on your left side, with your right hand down at your side.**

   See Steps 1 and 2 in the earlier section "The beginner clean" for full details on how to rack the kettlebell (refer to Figure 8-9b).

2. **With a tall spine, tighten your abs, pinch your glutes and lats, take a deep inhale, and press through your heels, keeping your knees locked as you forcefully exhale and press the kettlebell up so that your elbow is locked and your left bicep lines up with your left ear (see Figure 8-14).**

As you press the kettlebell up, rotate your palm slightly so that it's facing to the front in the top position. Typically, this rotation is quite natural for students, but it's worth noting that you won't press "straight" up from the rack position.

Tension equals force, so make a tight fist with your right hand, which is at your side, to help you press the kettlebell up.

3. **Still keeping your abs, glutes, and lats tight and your knees locked, in a controlled motion, actively bring the kettlebell back down into the left rack position.**

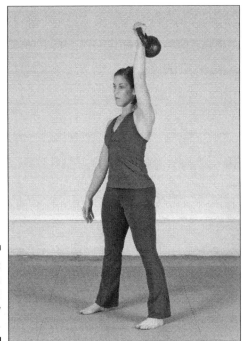

Figure 8-14:
The kettlebell military press.

Perform five repetitions on the left side; then take an extra swing to switch the kettlebell to the right side, clean the bell on the right side, and perform five repetitions of the military press on that side. (Use the alternating swing technique I describe in Chapter 6 to switch sides safely.)

Don't let your shoulder become disengaged from the lat muscle when pressing. Look in the mirror while pressing to see whether you're disengaging the shoulder from the lat — you know you're doing so if your shoulder is touching or close to touching your ear or if you feel like you're shrugging your shoulder.

Trying variations of the military press

Although infinite variations accompany most kettlebell exercises, I focus on the two main variations for the military press in this section: the push press and the clean and press.

The kettlebell push press

The *push press* gives your heart a little more cardio bump if you press with a lighter kettlebell. On the other hand, if you use a heavier bell than you normally would, the push press allows you to use more of your lower body to press the kettlebell up.

To do this exercise, follow these steps:

1. **Rack your kettlebell on your left side, with your right hand down at your side.**

   See Steps 1 and 2 in the earlier section "The beginner clean" for full details on how to perform this move (refer to Figure 8-9b).

2. **With a tall spine, tighten your abs, pinch your glutes and lats, take a deep inhale, and slightly push your hips back and bend your knees (see Figure 8-15).**

   Only push your hips back and bend your knees slightly in the push press. You aren't squatting in this exercise.

3. **As you forcefully exhale, press the kettlebell up, aggressively driving through your heels, locking out your knees, and tightening your legs, glutes, abs, and lats at the top (refer to Figure 8-14).**

   In the top position, your elbow is locked out, your left bicep lines up with your left ear, and your spine is tall and extended.

4. **Still keeping your abs, glutes, and lats tight and your knees locked, in a controlled motion, actively bring the kettlebell back down into the left rack position.**

Perform five repetitions on your left side; then take an extra swing to switch the kettlebell to the right side and perform five repetitions on that side. (Use the alternating swing technique I describe in Chapter 6 to switch sides safely.)

The kettlebell clean and press

The kettlebell *clean and press* adds a more dynamic element to the plain military press. The clean (which I describe earlier in this chapter) is typically thought of as a ballistic kettlebell exercise, while the military press is a grind movement. Put the two together and you have a very challenging exercise that literally works every major muscle group in your body.

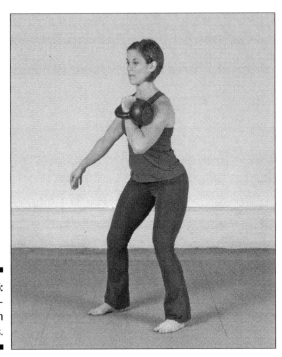

Figure 8-15:
The kettle-
bell push
press.

To do the clean and press, combine the kettlebell clean and the military press by following the earlier instructions for each exercise (see the sections "The clean" and "Doing the basic military press" and refer to Figures 8-10 and 8-14). Perform a clean, and, from the rack position, press the kettlebell up and bring it down to the rack position; then re-clean the bell and perform another press, repeating for five repetitions on each side. One complete clean and press equals one repetition.

With kettlebells, you're limited only by your imagination when it comes to variations of exercises. After you've mastered the clean and press, try some of the following more advanced variations (perform five repetitions of each):

✔ **The two-kettlebell military press:** Rack two kettlebells of the same size by following the instructions for the one-arm clean (see the section "The rack position") and then pressing both kettlebells up at the same time using the instructions I provide in the section "Doing the basic military press" as a guide.

✔ **The two-kettlebell push press:** Rack two kettlebells of the same size by following the instructions for the one-arm clean (see the section "The rack position") and then push pressing both bells up at the same time using the instructions I provide in the section "The kettlebell push press" as a guide.

- **The two-kettlebell clean and press:** Follow the instructions for the one-kettlebell clean and press that I describe earlier in this section. Use two kettlebells of the same size.

- **The alternating military press:** Rack two kettlebells of the same size (see the section "The rack position"). Then follow the instructions I provide in the section "Doing the basic military press" to press the bell on the left side, keeping the right kettlebell racked. Pull the left kettlebell down into the rack and keep it there; then press the right kettlebell up.

- **The seesaw press:** Use the instructions I provide in the section "The rack position" to rack two kettlebells of the same size. Press the left kettlebell up according to the instructions I provide in the section "Doing the basic military press," and actively pull the left kettlebell back down into the rack as you press the right kettlebell up.

Fixing bad military press form

The three most common military press–related errors for bad form that I observe with new students are

- Not keeping the shoulder in the lat muscle
- Not fully locking out the elbow at the top of the press
- Not bringing the arm back enough at the top of the press so the bicep is in line or close to being in line with the ear

You can resolve the first two errors by performing the corrective strategies I describe in Chapter 7, which focus on the same types of errors in form for the Turkish get-up. You can usually resolve the last error by looking in the mirror: As you perform the military press, look in a mirror to make sure your bicep is in line with your ear at the top of the press. Although I don't have any mirrors at my gym, sometimes a mirror can be really helpful — especially when I'm not there to guide you!

Practice the appropriate corrective strategies as you need to. Alternating between the corrective strategies and the actual military press will go a long way in keeping your form in check.

Chapter 9

Beginner Kettlebell Workouts to Lose the Jiggle and Build Strength

● ●

In This Chapter

▶ Going from flab to fab and feeling the cardio burn

▶ Working out with kettlebells for power and strength

▶ Setting up a weekly program of beginner workouts

● ●

*A*fter you have the basics of kettlebells down, it's time to put the exercises together into balanced and challenging workouts; lucky for you, this chapter is here to help you do just that. If you're focused on burning fat, Workouts 1 and 2 are great options to begin with. If you want to increase your lean muscle mass, power, and strength, Workout 3 is the right workout for you. Whatever your goals are, try all three workouts to see which ones you like best. Each workout is designed to work in combination with any of the others, so you can't go wrong no matter which way you decide to mix them up! (Flip to Chapter 18 for tips on setting and meeting your kettlebell fitness goals.)

Ideally, you'll perform the workouts in this chapter three to four days a week for about 25 to 30 minutes per workout. However, if you need to begin with only two days per week, you'll still see and feel results. The key is not to be intimidated — just pick one of the workouts and get started; after all, you'll feel better almost instantly after you begin. Just one workout has the power to energize you, improve your posture, and lower your stress levels. And don't forget to check out the information on setting up a weekly program at the end of this chapter; it'll guide you through your first month and help you stay motivated.

Use one kettlebell for the workouts, and make sure to have a good stopwatch handy to time your rest breaks. I offer a few active rest options to try out if you find that you don't need the rest breaks (Chapter 5 explains these active rest options in more detail); however, if you're using a challenging-enough size kettlebell, you should need the rest period for *at least* the time indicated in the workout (see Chapter 3 for choosing the right size kettlebell).

Master the techniques and exercises I describe in Chapters 4 through 8 before attempting any of the workouts in this chapter. Without a good foundation, you won't get the results you're looking for, and you could end up hurting yourself (ouch!).

Beginner Workout 1: Flab to Fab

Because the following workout uses all the basic exercises to keep your heart rate up, it's the perfect workout for the beginner who's focused on losing fat. The minimal rest breaks ensure that you'll stay in the fat-burning zone throughout the workout. In addition, the full-body exercises target all your muscle groups.

To warm up for this workout, do two or three dynamic stretches from Chapter 5 and three full Turkish get-ups on each side (see Chapter 7). After you're properly warmed up, follow the exercises listed in Table 9-1 to perform the flab-to-fab workout. If you decide to do the active rest options instead of taking the rest breaks, perform them for the same amount of time that's suggested for the rest breaks; refer to Chapter 5 for info on how to perform these active rest options properly.

Table 9-1	Beginner Flab-to-Fab Workout				
Exercise	*Number of Reps in Each Set*	*Number of Sets*	*Rest Period between Sets*	*Active Rest Option (Optional)*	*Reference Chapter*
Front squat with kettlebell held by the horns	10	1	30 seconds	Push-ups or plank	8
Two-arm swing	10	1	30 seconds	Burpees	6
Front squat with kettlebell racked on the left	5	1	10 seconds	---	8
Front squat with kettlebell racked on the right	5	1	10 seconds	---	8

Exercise	Number of Reps in Each Set	Number of Sets	Rest Period between Sets	Active Rest Option (Optional)	Reference Chapter
Alternating swing	20	1	30 seconds	Push-ups or burpees	6
Clean on the left	8	1	20 seconds	Jump squats	8
Clean on the right	8	1	20 seconds	Jump squats	8
Two-arm swing	10	1	30 seconds	Burpees	6
Clean/squat/ press combo on the left	10	2 (switch to right side before repeating set on left side)	30 seconds	Plank	9 (see the instruc- tions in this section)
Clean/squat/ press combo on the right	10	2 (switch to left side before repeating set on right side)	30 seconds	Plank	9 (see the instruc- tions in this section)
Push-up to T-hold on the left	3	2 (switch to right side before repeating set on left side)	30 seconds	---	5
Push-up to T-hold on the right	3	2 (switch to left side before repeating set on right side)	30 seconds	---	5

If you find you're too tired to complete the entire workout with good form, cut the number of all variations of the swing repetitions in half until you can work up to doing all the repetitions indicated in Table 9-1.

You may notice that I've included a combination of three separate exercises in this workout: the clean, the squat, and the press. As far as kettlebell combinations go, the *clean/squat/press combination* tops my list of favorites (along with the woman maker in Chapter 13). Whether I have 10 minutes to exercise or a full 30 minutes, I love combining these three moves. Sometimes I throw in some swings and rows for good measure, but even when I don't, this combo makes me feel as though I've worked all my major muscle groups and improved my cardiovascular endurance. If you're looking for the most bang for your buck, this combo will give it to you. (See Chapter 8 for detailed instructions on how to perform each individual exercise properly.) To do the combo, follow these steps:

1. **Stand with your feet shoulder width apart, your toes pointed forward, your arms down at your sides, and your kettlebell on the ground between your heels with the handle facing forward.**

2. **Sit back into your hips and reach down and back with your left arm to put your left hand on the kettlebell, taking care to keep your left arm close to your body; rotate your hand inward toward your bell so that your thumb is pointing backward (moving the kettlebell handle to face sideways as you do), and keep your right arm at your side.**

3. **Clean the kettlebell into the rack position on your left side by driving through your heels and snapping your hips to come up to standing, ending up with a tall spine and your right arm at your side (see Figure 9-1a).**

4. **With the kettlebell in the rack position, descend into the rock-bottom squat position by sitting back into your hips and bringing your rear end as close to the ground as you comfortably can while maintaining a neutral spine (see Figure 9-1b).**

   Your right arm should be out to your side when you're in the rock-bottom position.

5. **As you drive your heels through the ground to come up from the bottom of your squat, use your whole body to press the kettlebell up into a full lockout military press (see Figure 9-1c).**

   Don't wait until you stand up to press the bell; begin pressing it up as you come up from your squat by extending your left arm as you drive through your heels, locking out your elbow and keeping your left shoulder connected to the lat muscle at the top of the movement.

   The traditional military press is performed from the standing rack position, but this version is a push press, so you have to use your entire body to move the kettlebell by pressing the bell up into full lockout as you come up from your squat.

6. **Bring the kettlebell down into the rack position on the left side by repeating Step 3.**

To switch to the right side, you can either set the kettlebell down and clean it into the rack on the right side or take an extra (alternating) swing to switch and clean it on the right side from the backswing position. See Chapter 6 for details on how to do the alternating swing.

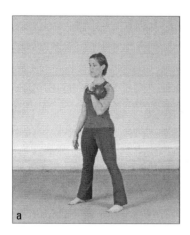 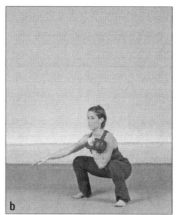

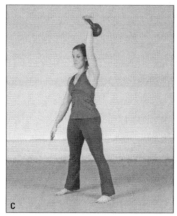

Figure 9-1:
The clean/
squat/press
combination.

After you complete all the moves in Table 9-1, cool down with any three stretches or Z-Health movements from Chapter 5.

Beginner Workout 2: Cardio Burn

This lung-searing workout is great for beginners who want to increase their cardiovascular endurance because it involves performing a squat/lunge/ press combination after each set of swings. This seemingly simple workout will have you gasping for air throughout the workout because swings take a tremendous amount of cardiovascular capacity. When you couple them with a challenging combo like the squat/lunge/press, you get an even greater cardio burn.

REMEMBER

To warm up for this workout, do two or three dynamic stretches from Chapter 5. After your warm-up, follow the exercises listed in Table 9-2 to perform the cardio-burn workout.

For this workout, don't set down the kettlebell until you reach one of the rest periods indicated in Table 9-2.

Table 9-2		Beginner Cardio-Burn Workout			
Exercise	*Number of Reps in Each Set*	*Number of Sets*	*Rest Period between Sets*	*Active Rest Option (Optional)*	*Reference Chapter*
One-arm swing on the left	5	1	---	---	6
Squat/lunge/ press combo on the left	5	1	---	---	9 (see the instructions in this section)
One-arm swing on the right	5	1	---	---	6
Squat/lunge/ press combo on the right	5	1	1 minute	---	9 (see the instructions in this section)
One-arm swing on the left	8	1	---	---	6
Squat/lunge/ press combo on the left	8	1	---	---	9 (see the instructions in this section)
One-arm swing on the right	8	1	---	---	6
Squat/lunge/ press combo on the right	8	1	1 minute	---	9 (see the instructions in this section)
One-arm swing on the left	10	1	---	---	6
Squat/lunge/ press combo on the left	10	1	---	---	9 (see the instructions in this section)
One-arm swing on the right	10	1	---	---	6
Squat/lunge/ press combo on the right	10	1	1 minute	---	9 (see the instructions in this section)

As I do in the flab-to-fab workout earlier in this chapter, I include a combination of three separate exercises in the cardio-burn workout. This time, the combo consists of the squat from Chapter 8, the lunge (a basic fitness move), and the press from Chapter 8. Follow these steps to do the *squat/lunge/press combination:*

1. **Stand with your feet shoulder width apart, your toes pointed forward, your arms down at your sides, and your kettlebell on the ground between your heels with the handle facing forward.**

2. **Sit back into your hips and reach down and back with your left arm to put your left hand on the kettlebell, taking care to keep your left arm close to your body; rotate your hand inward toward your bell so that your thumb is pointing backward (moving the kettlebell handle to face sideways as you do), and keep your right arm at your side.**

3. **Clean the kettlebell into the rack position on your left side by driving through your heels and snapping your hips to come up to standing, ending up with a tall spine and your right arm at your side (refer to Figure 9-1a).**

4. **With the kettlebell in the rack position, descend into the rock-bottom squat position by sitting back into your hips and bringing your rear end as close to the ground as you comfortably can while maintaining a neutral spine (see Figure 9-2a).**

   Your right arm should be out to your side when you're in the rock-bottom position.

5. **Without pausing in the rock-bottom position, drive up through your heels, keeping your knees and core stable, to the fully standing position that I describe in Step 1; make sure your spine is tall, and pinch your glutes at the top of the movement.**

6. **Step back into a lunge position with your left leg, letting your right knee bend as you do so; keep your spine tall and your abs tight (see Figure 9-2b).**

7. **Press through your right heel to stand back up tall, bringing your feet together.**

8. **Perform a military press with your left arm, making sure to lock out your elbow (see Figure 9-2c).**

Squat and lunge with the kettlebell racked on the side indicated in Table 9-2, and don't press the bell up until you've stood up from the lunge. Why? As a beginner, you probably lack the core stability to perform the press as you're coming up from the lunge (which is a more advanced combo) and could end up injuring yourself.

All done with the moves in Table 9-2? Great! Cool down with any three stretches or Z-Health movements from Chapter 5.

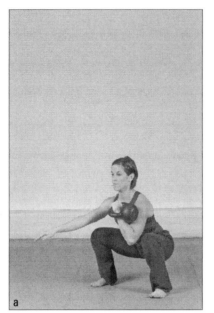
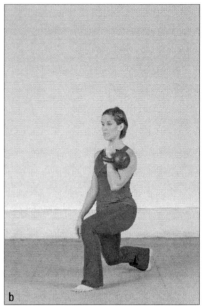
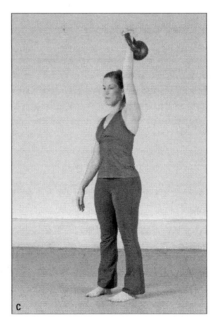

Figure 9-2:
The squat/
lunge/press
combination.

Beginner Workout 3: Power and Strength

With the power-and-strength workout, you perform low reps with lots of rest in between sets. But don't think this workout is any easier than the others! This workout is best when you're ready to move up to a heavier kettlebell and are interested in gaining more power and strength from your kettlebell workouts, but it's also a good balance for your fat-burning and cardio/endurance-building workouts. And don't worry — just because you're using heavier weight and building strength doesn't mean you're going to get big, bulky muscles.

To warm up for this workout, do two or three dynamic stretches or Z-Health options from Chapter 5. Then do ten single reps of full Turkish get-ups (*single reps* means you switch sides after each rep). After you're done with your warm-up, follow the exercises listed in Table 9-3 to perform the power-and-strength workout.

For this workout, you can either finish the reps and sets indicated for each exercise before moving on to the next exercise or complete one set of each exercise and move on to the next, repeating this cycle four times and completing four total sets for each exercise.

Table 9-3	Beginner Power-and-Strength Workout				
Exercise	**Number of Reps in Each Set**	**Number of Sets**	**Rest Period between Sets**	**Active Rest Option (Optional)**	**Reference Chapter**
Clean/squat combo on the left	5	4	1 minute	Push-ups	9 (see the instructions in this section)
Clean/squat combo on the right	5	4	1 minute	Push-ups	9 (see the instructions in this section)
Military press on the left	5	4	1 minute	Push-up to T-hold	8
Military press on the right	5	4	1 minute	Push-up to T-hold	8
Burpees	20	4	1 minute	Push-ups	5

As I do in the workouts in Tables 9-1 and 9-2, I include a combination of exercises in this workout, but this time I use only two exercises in the combo: the clean and the squat (both from Chapter 8). Follow these steps to do the *clean/ squat combination:*

1. **Stand with your feet shoulder width apart, your toes pointed forward, your arms down at your sides, and your kettlebell on the ground between your heels with the handle facing forward.**

2. **Sit back into your hips and reach down and back with your left arm to put your left hand on the kettlebell, taking care to keep your left arm close to your body; rotate your hand inward toward your bell so that your thumb is pointing backward (moving the kettlebell handle to face sideways as you do), and keep your right arm at your side.**

3. **Clean the kettlebell into the rack position on your left side by driving through your heels and snapping your hips to come up to standing, ending up with a tall spine and your right arm at your side (refer to Figure 9-1a).**

4. **With the kettlebell in the rack position, descend into the rock-bottom squat position by sitting back into your hips and bringing your rear end as close to the ground as you comfortably can while maintaining a neutral spine (refer to Figure 9-1b).**

   Your right arm should be out to your side when you're in the rock-bottom position.

5. **Without pausing in the rock-bottom position, drive up through your heels, keeping your knees and core stable, to the fully standing position I describe in Step 1; make sure your spine is tall, and pinch your glutes at the top of the movement.**

After you're finished with your workout, cool down with any three stretches or Z-Health movements from Chapter 5.

Putting Together a Program of Beginner Workouts during the Week

You may be wondering how to put the workouts from the previous sections together into one cohesive training program. Although the task of creating your own training program may seem daunting, you need to take some time to do so. After all, having a plan of action is essential to finding success in any workout program. Use the sample plans I offer in the following sections to guide you in formulating your workout program.

Begin by choosing how many days per week you can reasonably fit exercise into your schedule. (The best thing about the workouts in this chapter is that they're short but intense, so if you have only an hour a week to work out, you can do so effectively.) After you choose how many days you're going to work out, stick to the program for four weeks. After you complete a four-week cycle, focus on the advanced exercises I cover in Part III of this book, and then continue with the advanced workout plans in Chapter 13.

Kettlebell training is a complete cardio and strength-training tool, and, if you're using the correct size kettlebell (see Chapter 3 for pointers on picking the right size for you), you shouldn't feel the need to engage in any other weight-training or cardio program. Of course, exceptions to this rule are out there — perhaps you're a runner or cyclist who wants to use kettlebells to improve your performance in your sport. In that case, refer to Chapter 16 for the appropriate workout mix. For most kettlebellers, however, any other physical activity you do in addition to your kettlebell routine should be complimentary. In other words, don't overtrain your body by doing too much — if you do, you'll end up with marginal results and very little long-term benefit. Some great complimentary programs to kettlebells include physical programs, such as Pilates or yoga, and body weight–training programs (programs that use only your body weight for resistance). If you're interested in such programs, check out *Yoga For Dummies,* 2nd Edition, by Georg Feuerstein and Larry Payne and *Pilates For Dummies* by Ellie Herman, both published by Wiley.

A sample plan for doing kettlebells two days per week

If you have only two days per week to workout using kettlebells, ideally you'd put one day of rest in between your workouts. In addition, you want to choose a different emphasis for each workout so that you have a balanced workout routine. For example, you could do a fat-burning workout on your first workout day and a cardio/endurance-building workout on your second workout day. A two-days-a-week plan like the one that follows is perfect for those of you who are new to exercise or who participate in other fitness programs, like yoga or Pilates:

Tuesday

Beginner Workout 1

Thursday

Beginner Workout 2

If you opt for the two-days-a-week kettlebell routine, try to be active at least two other days each week. Pilates, yoga, and body weight exercises are great options, but any other physical activities you enjoy are good, too.

A sample plan for doing kettlebells three days per week

If you can fit in three kettlebell workouts per week, try to put a day in between each workout. If you need to put two workout days back to back, though, don't worry. Just remember to adjust the emphasis and intensity accordingly. For example, if you end up having to workout two days in a row, don't do a cardio/endurance-building workout on both of those days. Instead, choose a cardio/endurance-building or fat-burning workout and a power-and-strength type of workout to vary the emphasis and intensity. A three-days-a-week kettlebell workout like the one that follows is best for someone who is regularly active. But even if you do exercise regularly, expect some soreness your first few weeks until your body adjusts to the frequency of your kettle-bell workouts.

Monday	*Wednesday*	*Friday*
Beginner Workout 1	Beginner Workout 2	Beginner Workout 3

If you opt for the three-days-a-week kettlebell routine, try to be active at least one other day each week. Pilates, yoga, and body weight exercises are great options, but any other physical activities you enjoy are good, too.

A sample plan for doing kettlebells four days per week

Practicing kettlebell workouts four days per week takes dedication, but the results come even faster than if you worked out only two or three days per week. With a four-days-a-week workout, you end up doing a back-to-back workout, which is totally fine as long as you vary the type and intensity of workouts you do so that you don't end up overdoing it. For example, you can do your fat-burning workout on Monday and your power-and-strength work-out on Tuesday, take Wednesday as a recovery day, change the emphasis on Thursday to a cardio/endurance-building workout, take another day of recov-ery on Friday, and finish the week with your fat-burning workout. Of course, your particular workout routine depends on your goals, but these general guidelines can help you get started. A four-days-a-week plan like the following one is best for someone who has worked through the three-days-a-week workout plan for at least a few weeks:

Monday	*Tuesday*	*Thursday*	*Saturday*
Beginner Workout 1	Beginner Workout 3	Beginner Workout 2	Beginner Workout 1

If you opt for the four-days-a-week kettlebell routine, try to be active at least one other day each week. Pilates, yoga, and body weight exercises are great options, but any other physical activities you enjoy are good, too.

Part III
Mastering Advanced Kettlebell Moves

The 5th Wave   By Rich Tennant

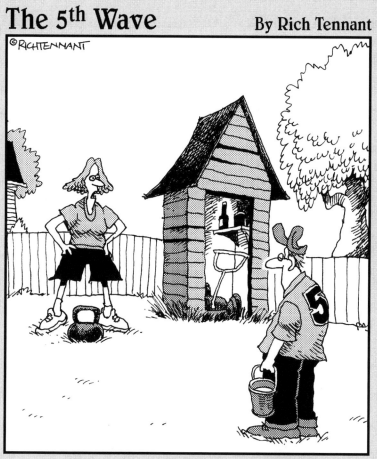

"I'm starting with the swinging moves. In doing so, I hope to strengthen my core, burn calories, and knock down this shed."

In this part . . .

The exercises and workout routines in this part are for those of you who are ready to take on more advanced kettlebell moves. Here, you discover some exercises that help you gain strength, flexibility, and mobility and other exercises that are specifically designed to strengthen your core; all these advanced moves help add variety to your regular kettlebell routine. I also include the five best advanced kettlebell exercises to do if you're ready to take your training up a notch.

The advanced kettlebell workouts I cover in this part are guaranteed to get your heart rate up. If you're really up for a challenge, try out the highly effective kettlebell combination exercises that are sure to work every muscle in your body — even the ones you didn't know you had!

Chapter 10

Kettlebell Exercises to Help You Gain Strength, Flexibility, and Mobility

* *

In This Chapter

▶ Warming up with the windmill

▶ Working your upper body with different types of rows

▶ Building your overall strength with the high pull

▶ Getting a great lower body with the single-leg dead lift, tactical lunge, and deck squat

* *

After you master the foundational kettlebell exercises in Part II, you can focus on the exercises in this chapter, which help you develop strength, flexibility, and mobility. By the time you're done, you'll have worked all your major muscle groups, including your arms, chest, back, core, and legs.

I recommend taking the two exercises you like the best from this chapter and incorporating them into your foundational program. For example, the windmill and single-leg dead lift would be perfect additions to a swing, clean, press, and squat routine. You can also add in one of the row variations for an even more complete program.

The Windmill

The windmill is one of my favorite full-body exercises. Like the Turkish get-up in Chapter 7, the windmill packs a powerful punch without requiring very many repetitions. It works your core and shoulders and increases mobility in your hips and shoulders; not to mention, you get a really nice stretch, too.

As a beginner, you want to use the windmill as a warm-up exercise because, like the Turkish get-up, the windmill requires you to hold the kettlebell over your head for a period of time. If you're fatigued, your chances of performing the exercise incorrectly or having to bail out on a repetition increase. Quality of repetitions is much more important than quantity. Indeed, you get much more from performing one good repetition than you get from performing ten bad ones, so keep this exercise at the beginning of your routine until you become a more proficient kettlebeller — at which time you can add the windmill into your routine anywhere you see fit.

I describe the three main windmill variations in the following sections: the low windmill, the high windmill, and the two-kettlebell windmill. It's essential to start with the low windmill to make sure you have the right amount of mobility to perform the high windmill. Typically, students who lack mobility and flexibility in their hips and shoulders can't perform the high windmill with good enough form for the exercise to be of any benefit to them. If you lack mobility in your shoulders or hips, practice the low windmill and the corrective exercise that I describe later in the "Correcting your windmill form with a partner exercise" section before incorporating the high windmill into your workout. After you master both the low windmill and the high windmill, you can challenge yourself with the two-kettlebell windmill.

Keep your elbow locked and your eye on the kettlebell at all times throughout every variation of the windmill. If there's a break in your elbow or if you look elsewhere during the exercise, you won't be able to control the kettlebell and you can injure yourself.

Make sure you know how to both clean and press the kettlebell properly (see Chapter 8) before you try out any variation of the windmill. You absolutely have to know how to clean and press a kettlebell to perform the windmill safely and correctly.

The low windmill

The *low windmill* introduces your body to the windmill movement without having you put the kettlebell overhead just yet. Pushing into your hips as you perform this movement is the key to doing it right, so take your time as you move through the low windmill and really feel how to push into the hips properly. To do the low windmill, follow these steps:

1. **Stand with your feet shoulder width apart, your arms at your sides, and your kettlebell on the ground between your feet with the handle facing forward; then turn both your feet 45 degrees to the right.**

2. **Raise your left arm above you, keeping your eyes on your left hand as you push your left hip out and back.**

3. **Slowly descend, continuing to push into your left hip and keeping your head in line with your spine; find the kettlebell handle with your right hand (see Figure 10-1a).**

   Make sure to keep your left arm straightened and your left elbow locked above you. If you need to bend your right knee slightly as you descend, feel free to do so; just make sure to push into the left hip as you bend your knee instead of shifting your weight forward into your right leg. Keep your left leg straightened.

4. **Pick the kettlebell off the floor with your right hand, and, with your right arm straightened, glide it along your right leg as you drive through your heels and stand up tall, pinching your glutes and abs (see Figure 10-1b).**

   Your eyes are still on your left hand, and your left elbow is still locked. Don't shrug your shoulders at the top of the movement; keep your shoulders down and away from your ears so that you keep a long spine throughout the movement.

Do four repetitions on the left side without setting down the kettlebell; then set the bell down, switch sides, and repeat for four repetitions on the right side.

Think about opening your chest and opening the shoulder of the arm that's raised above you as you perform any variation of the windmill.

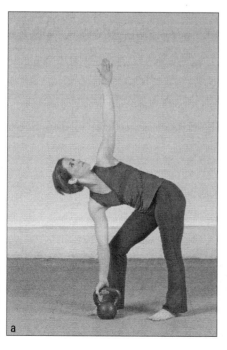
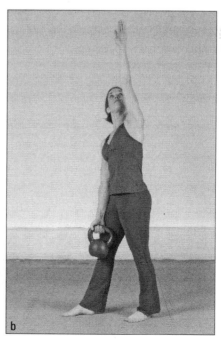

Figure 10-1:
The low
windmill.

a   b

The high windmill

The *high windmill* challenges your core stability and flexibility more than the low windmill because it involves performing the movement with the kettlebell overhead. To do the high windmill, follow these steps:

1. **Stand with your feet shoulder width apart, your toes pointed forward, your arms down at your sides, and your kettlebell on the ground between your heels with the handle facing forward.**

2. **Get into the rack position on the left side by sitting back into your hips, picking up the kettlebell with both hands, and then bringing the kettlebell snug up to your chest as you stand back up; then turn both of your feet 45 degrees to the right.**

   See Chapter 8 for all the details on how to get into the rack position.

3. **Press the kettlebell up with your left hand, keeping your eyes on the kettlebell and your left shoulder engaged in its socket.**

   See Chapter 8 for details on how to press the kettlebell.

4. **Push into your left hip as you slowly descend, keeping your left leg straight and bending your right knee slightly if needed; keep your head in line with your spine as you reach for the middle of your foot with your right hand, and then tap the floor with your right hand (see Figure 10-2a).**

   Keep your left arm straightened and your elbow locked during this movement, and don't shift your weight forward into your right leg.

   The windmill isn't a side bend. Think about pushing your hip out as if you were going to bump someone with your hip, and continue pushing into the hip as you descend.

   You may be unable to reach the ground with your fingertips, which is perfectly fine; as long as you're close, you still benefit from the exercise.

5. **Drive through your heels, and, in a controlled motion, stand up tall, still keeping your eyes on the kettlebell and your left elbow locked and pinching your glutes and abs (see Figure 10-2b).**

Repeat for a total of four repetitions on the left side without bringing the kettlebell back into the rack position; then switch sides by racking the kettlebell on the right side and perform four repetitions on that side.

If you're having trouble performing the high windmill with your feet facing 45 degrees, point your toes straight ahead and see whether that change makes a difference in your form. You still need to push into the hip, but now you can visualize pushing both your hips back toward the wall, while leading with the hip of the arm that's extended. In addition, you can try having the foot of the extended arm facing forward, while the other is at 45 degrees. Either of these options is acceptable, so use whichever one works best for you.

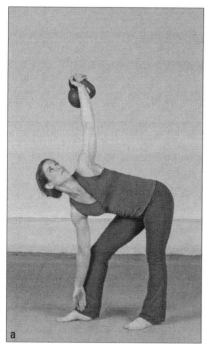
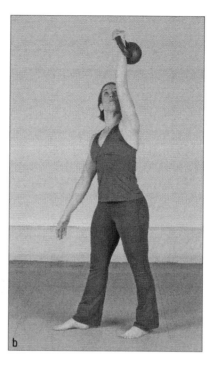

Figure 10-2:
The high
windmill.

You can let your front knee (the one opposite your extended arm) bend slightly as you descend. However, you must make sure that you shift your weight back into the hip of the arm that's extended as the knee is bending. All too often students bend the front knee and then shift their weight forward into it — which is wrong. You won't get any benefit from the windmill if you perform it this way.

The two-kettlebell windmill

Although the high windmill should be challenging when you use an appropriately sized kettlebell (see Chapter 3 for details on picking the right size), adding another kettlebell to the exercise gives your body another dimension of difficulty. To do the *two-kettlebell windmill,* you can use two kettlebells of the same size, or, if you lack flexibility and mobility, you can use a very light kettlebell in the high position and use a heavier one for the low position. It's your call!

To perform the two-kettlebell windmill, follow these steps:

1. **Stand with your feet shoulder width apart, your toes pointed forward, your arms down at your sides, and your kettlebells on the ground between your heels with the handles facing forward.**

2. **Get into the rack position on the left side, and have your second kettlebell resting on the ground between your feet; then turn both of your feet 45 degrees to the right.**

   See Chapter 8 for details on how to get into the rack position.

3. **Press up the racked kettlebell with your left hand, keeping your eyes on the bell.**

   See Chapter 8 for details on how to press the kettlebell.

4. **Push into your left hip as you slowly descend, keeping your left leg straight and bending your right knee slightly if needed; keeping your head in line with your spine, reach for the kettlebell that's at your feet with your right hand (see Figure 10-3a).**

   Keep your left arm straightened and your elbow locked during this movement.

5. **After you find the kettlebell handle, pick it up off the ground, keeping your right arm straightened and spine neutral; drive through your heels, and, in a controlled motion, stand up tall, keeping the left elbow locked and your eyes on the kettlebell above you (see Figure 10-3b).**

   Be sure to pinch your glutes and abs during this movement.

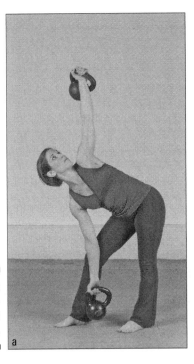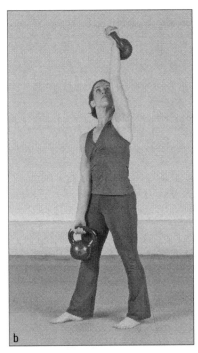

Figure 10-3:
The two-kettlebell windmill.

Perform a total of four repetitions on the left side without setting either kettlebell down; then switch sides by racking the kettlebell on the right side and perform four repetitions on that side.

Correcting your windmill form with a partner exercise

Some students find the windmill difficult to perform if they don't have the hip and shoulder flexibility to execute the movement with good form. The partner exercise I describe in this section helps you get your hips to move properly for the windmill and, by default, helps you keep your chest and working shoulder open during the movement.

To do this corrective exercise, you need a jump rope, large strap, or stretch band. A very large beach towel may also work. Follow these steps to do this partner exercise:

1. **Start with your feet shoulder width apart, and have an imaginary kettlebell racked on the left side.**

2. **Have your partner stand behind you and hold the jump rope or band around your hips with both hands (see Figure 10-4a).**

   Holding the band around your hips means placing it in the crease your legs would make if you sat down in a chair.

3. **Press your imaginary kettlebell up with your left hand.**

4. **As you push into your left hip to descend, have your partner gently pull on the rope or band to guide your hips back.**

5. **Reach for the ground with your right hand, keeping your eye on your imaginary bell as your partner continues to gently guide your hips back with the rope or band (see Figure 10-4b).**

6. **As your partner slowly releases the pressure on your hips, drive through your heels and stand up tall, pinching your glutes and abs at the top.**

   Keep your left arm straightened and your elbow locked during this movement.

Repeat for a total of five repetitions on your left side; then switch sides and repeat for five repetitions on your right side.

After you've practiced this corrective technique, attempt the high windmill with a very light kettlebell and see whether your form has improved.

You can have your partner assist you with the rope or band with the kettlebell in the low position, but don't attempt to have them assist you with the kettlebell in the high position. Doing so could put you both at risk for injury.

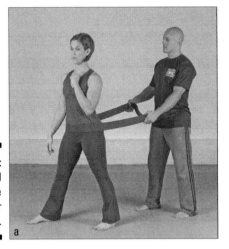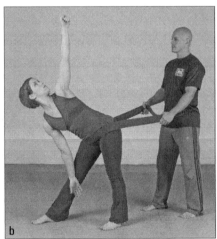

Figure 10-4:
A windmill
corrective
partner
exercise.

 If you still need to work on shoulder flexibility, practice the Turkish get-up in Chapter 7, and refer to the corrective techniques for the military press in Chapter 8.

The One-Arm Row

The *one-arm kettlebell row* is very similar to the one-arm row you do with a dumbbell. But because the weight of a kettlebell is distributed much differently than the weight of a dumbbell, you feel this exercise not only in your back muscles but also in your abdominals, arms, and shoulders.

The row is considered a *pull exercise* (one in which you pull a kettlebell or your body weight toward you). You should have at least one pull exercise in your kettlebell workout routine because it balances nicely with the squat and other *push exercises* (ones in which you push the bell away from you) that you do. To round out your routine, you can alternate between the one-arm row, pull-ups, and the renegade row with two kettlebells (see Chapter 11), or you can stick with the one-arm row and one-arm renegade row variations I describe in this chapter.

 As you perform the row, keep your eyes on the bell, or look 6 feet in front of you and down so that your spine stays neutral and you don't strain your neck during the exercise.

To do the one-arm row, follow these steps:

1. **Stand with your feet shoulder width apart, your arms at your sides, and your kettlebell between your feet, handle facing sideways.**

2. **Bend your right knee, and step back on a slight outward angle with your left leg, keeping the left heel down and left foot angled slightly; rest your right elbow on your right knee, and have your kettlebell next to the inside of your right foot (see Figure 10-5a).**

   Don't step straight back into a lunge (do so at an angle), and make sure your left leg is straightened behind you.

3. **Place your left hand on the kettlebell handle; keeping the kettlebell close to the rib cage, pull back toward your hip as you concentrate on crushing the handle of the bell (see Figure 10-5b).**

   Keep your abs tight and your shoulders square throughout the movement.

4. **Return the kettlebell to the ground without taking your hand off the handle.**

Repeat for eight repetitions on the left side; then switch sides and perform eight repetitions on the right side.

Figure 10-5: The one-arm kettlebell row.

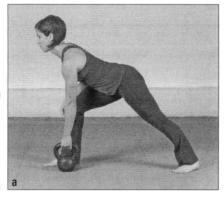 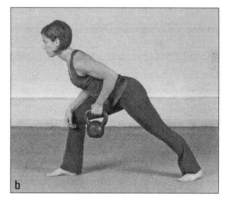

a   b

You can make a fist with your free hand as you perform the row to remind your body to keep tension — after all, tension equals force. Also, keep your shoulders square and don't raise your working shoulder out of the socket while performing the one-arm row.

The Renegade Row with One Kettlebell

The *renegade row with one kettlebell* challenges your ability to keep yourself stable by using your abdominals and back muscles. It also prepares you for the more challenging and difficult renegade row with two kettlebells, which I describe in Chapter 11.

I remember when I was a traditional weight lifter and I was asked by a former trainer to do the renegade row with a dumbbell. At the time, I considered myself strong and fit, but I was quite humbled when I attempted to do the renegade row. I nearly fell over because my body was not yet trained to know how to work as one unit. Chances are you'll feel like you're about to fall over while doing the row portion of the renegade row — but don't worry. Just do a couple of reps until you feel more stable and build up your core strength to be able to do ten repetitions per side with control and stability.

To do the renegade row, follow these steps:

1. **Get into a push-up position with your kettlebell positioned on the ground next to your left hand.**

   You can be in either a traditional push-up position in which your hands are about shoulder width apart, your shoulders are over your wrists, and your legs are slightly wider than your shoulders, or in a less traditional position on your knees with your hands about shoulder width apart and your shoulders over your wrists.

2. **As you place your left hand on your kettlebell, stabilize yourself by bracing your abs and tightening your glutes (see Figure 10-6a).**

   You can use another kettlebell turned on its side with its handle facing away from you to help stabilize you (use the extra bell on the side opposite your working arm). If you don't have another kettlebell, use a dumbbell. You can also spread your legs to form a wide base for more stability.

3. **Pull the kettlebell toward your rib cage, still keeping your abs braced and your thighs and glutes tight (see Figure 10-6b).**

4. **With precision and control, return the bell to the ground.**

Perform five repetitions on your left side; then switch sides and perform five repetitions on your right side.

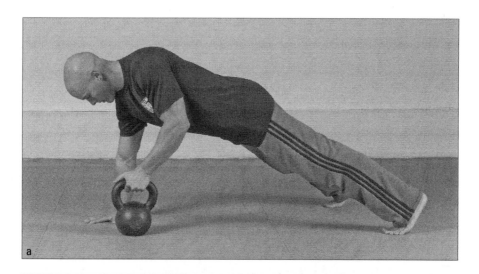

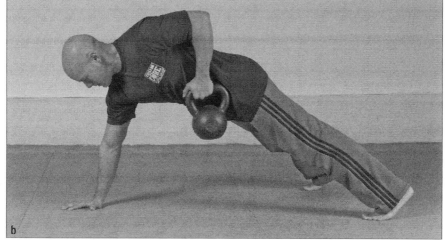

Figure 10-6:
The
renegade
row with
one kettle-
bell.

The High Pull

The *high pull* is another kettlebell exercise that works a majority of your major muscle groups; it also prepares you to perform the snatch (see Chapter 12 for more on that exercise). The high pull's dynamic motion can be a bit tricky to understand at first, but it's worth taking the time to learn because doing so improves your chances of snatching well. (And the snatch is a quintessential kettlebell exercise that you must make a part of your routine because the benefits you get from it are tremendous.)

You can perform the high pull a couple of different ways, but the method I show you in this section is the most basic and emphasizes the chest and back; it's the best variation to prepare you for the snatch.

The principles you master in the swing (Chapter 6) and the clean (Chapter 8) come into play for the high pull, so take a look at both of those chapters before you try the high pull.

To do the high pull, follow these steps:

1. **Stand with your feet shoulder width apart, your weight in your heels, your arms down at your sides, and your kettlebell resting on the ground between your feet with the handle facing forward.**

2. **Sit back into your hips and put your left hand on the kettlebell and your right arm out to the side (see Figure 10-7a).**

   See Chapter 4 for details on how to sit back into your hips properly.

3. **Drive through your heels and snap your hips to stand up and bring the kettlebell off the ground; in one fluid motion, pull the kettlebell toward your chest, tightening your glutes and abs at the top of the movement.**

   Your hip snap initiates the pull of the exercise. To continue the pull back toward your chest, bend your left elbow and pull your arm back as if you want to strike something behind you so that the bottom of the kettlebell is facing outward (see Figure 10-7b).

4. **Let the kettlebell come back to the backswing position by punching it slightly forward and toward the ground (see Figure 10-7c).**

Don't hesitate at the top of the pull or the kettlebell will end up flopping down. In addition, don't twist your waist at the top of the pull; keep your shoulders square. The high pull is a rapid, ballistic movement, so you need to move and control the bell using your hip snap, just like in the swing or clean.

Keep your working (left) shoulder in the socket and away from your ear during the movement. Tighten your working lat muscle, abs, and glutes so that you control the kettlebell completely throughout the movement.

Perform eight repetitions on the left side, and then set the kettlebell down or take an extra swing to switch sides (see Chapter 6 for more on the alternating swing); perform eight repetitions on that side.

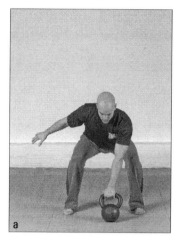
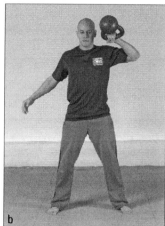
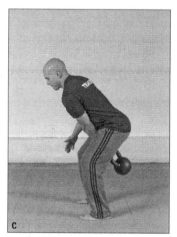

Figure 10-7:
The high
pull.

If the high pull gives you trouble, turn to Chapter 6 to go through the steps for the swing and Chapter 8 to go through the steps for the clean and press. The concepts and techniques that help you practice those exercises apply to the high pull, too.

If you're comfortable doing the high pull with one kettlebell, you can add a second bell to spice things up a bit. To do a *double-kettlebell high pull,* use two kettlebells of the same size and follow the steps for the single-kettlebell high pull. Make sure you're proficient with one bell before attempting to use two.

The Single-Leg Dead Lift

If you don't have good balance, the *single-leg dead lift* is an excellent exercise to add to your kettlebell routine. In addition to improving your balance, this exercise gives your lower-body workout routine a lift, providing your muscle groups (especially your glutes and legs) with a variety you don't get from doing squats alone.

In the following sections, I explain how to do the single-leg dead lift with two hands on the kettlebell and how to perform a one-handed variation of the lift. I also describe a useful corrective exercise if you're having trouble with your lift form.

Use correct breathing techniques to protect your lower back and to keep you stable throughout all versions of the single-leg dead lift. Make sure to inhale before you descend and exhale while you drive back up to the top position. (See Chapter 5 for more on breathing right during your kettlebell exercises.)

Doing the single-leg dead lift with two hands on the kettlebell

The single-leg dead lift with a kettlebell is an exercise that not only strengthens your legs and glutes but also builds your core stability and balance. To do the single-leg dead lift with two hands on the kettlebell, follow these steps:

1. **Stand with your feet slightly apart and your arms down in front of your thighs; hold your kettlebell with both hands.**

2. **Lift your left leg off the ground and behind you, take a deep inhale through your nose, and look 6 feet in front of you and down at a focal point (see Figure 10-8a).**

3. **Slowly sit back into your hips and descend as you let the right knee bend slightly and the kettlebell follow your movement (see Figure 10-8b); gently touch the ground with your bell if your flexibility and balance allow you to do so.**

See Chapter 4 for more on how to sit back into your hips.

Keep your spine neutral as you push as far back into your hips as you can. Make sure to maintain complete balance and stability throughout the movement.

4. In a controlled movement, drive through your right heel as you exhale and stand up tall with your abs and glutes pinched.

Place your left foot back on the ground as you come up only if you're coming off balance and need to reset yourself. Otherwise, keep the left leg off the ground until you've completed all your repetitions on the left side.

Perform eight repetitions on the left side; then switch sides and perform eight repetitions on the right side. ***Note:*** When you switch sides, take the time to set down the kettlebell first. You don't want to risk dropping the bell on your foot — ouch!

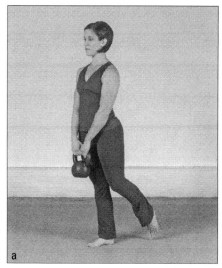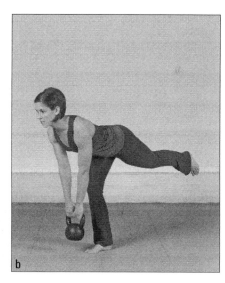

Figure 10-8:
The single-leg dead lift.

Your hips lead the race for most kettlebell exercises, including the single-leg dead lift. Push back into your hips first, and let the working knee follow your hips. If you feel the single-leg dead lift mostly in your glutes and hamstrings, you're doing it right. If you feel it mostly in your thighs, you're performing something more like a single-leg squat (which is a different exercise with a different emphasis; see Chapter 12 for details on the single-leg squat or pistol exercise).

If you feel the single-leg dead lift in your back, skip ahead to the corrective technique outlined in the "Performing a corrective exercise for the single-leg dead lift" section later in this chapter. If you don't correct your form before trying the one-handed single-leg dead lift, you risk injury.

Trying a one-handed variation of the single-leg dead lift

Although it's typically easier for first-time students to perform the single-leg dead lift with two hands on the kettlebell, you can also do this exercise with only one hand on the bell. You undoubtedly feel less stable during this variation because your body is forced to balance and compensate for the weight being concentrated on one side. If you're already balance challenged, practice the two-handed version for now and check out the corrective technique in the next section. For those of you who can perform the two-handed variation with good form, why not try the one-handed version?

To do the *one-handed single-leg dead lift,* follow the steps for the two-handed variation in the preceding section, except place the kettlebell in the hand corresponding to your working leg (the one you're balancing on). In Figure 10-9, the model is holding the kettlebell in her left hand and standing on her left leg. Perform eight repetitions on each side.

If you've become proficient at both variations of the single-leg dead lift, try holding the kettlebell in the hand opposite your working leg (contra lateral) or use two kettlebells of the same size, one in each hand.

Performing a corrective exercise for the single-leg dead lift

If you feel any pain in your lower back during the single-leg dead lift, you're most likely folding over at the hips rather than sitting back into the hips. Chapter 4 thoroughly discusses how to properly sit back into the hips, so flip to that chapter to reference the information you need. After doing so, try the corrective exercise I describe in this section.

You should never feel any pain in your lower back during kettlebell exercises. If you do, turn to Chapter 4 to perfect the movement of sitting back into your hips and maintaining a neutral spine.

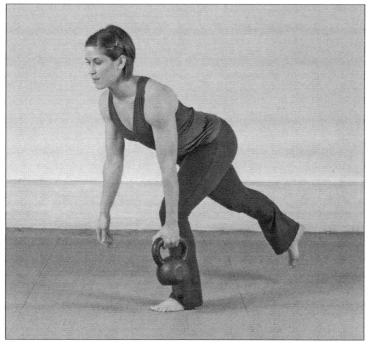

Figure 10-9:
The one-handed single-leg dead lift.

To make sure you're sitting back into your hips to perform the single-leg dead lift, try this simple corrective exercise, for which you need to use the back of a chair and a mirror. To do this corrective exercise, follow these steps:

1. **Place your chair in front of a mirror so you can see yourself from a side view.**

2. **Place one hand on the chair back and get into the single-leg dead lift start position I describe in Step 1 in the earlier section "Doing the single-leg dead lift with two hands on the kettlebell," but don't use your kettlebell.**

3. **Follow Steps 2 through 4 for the single-leg dead lift I describe in the earlier section, but pause when you have pushed as far back into your hips as you can and look in the mirror.**

    Does your spine have a nice natural *S* curve (see Figure 10-10), or is it rounded? If it's rounded, practice reaching back into your hips (a movement I outline in Chapter 4).

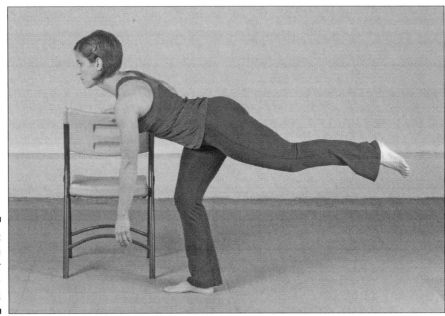

Figure 10-10: A corrective exercise for the single-leg dead lift.

I've encountered many students who have great swing form and understand how to sit back into their hips, yet they can't apply it to the single-leg dead lift — even though it's essentially the same movement. The only difference is you're balancing on one leg. Remember to let the hips lead you back and to go slow so that you can concentrate on your form. After you're comfortable with your form using the chair, perform this chair-corrective technique again, but, this time, use your kettlebell.

The Tactical Lunge

The *tactical lunge* adds some fun to the traditional lunge. Like the traditional lunge, the tactical lunge targets your legs and glutes, but, as an added bonus, the tactical lunge really taxes your stabilizer muscles (your core) and challenges your balance. In this kettlebell exercise, you pass the bell under your leg from one hand to the other as you lunge.

To do the tactical lunge, follow these steps:

1. **Stand with your feet a few inches apart and hold the kettlebell with two hands, keeping your arms down in front of your body.**

2. **Step back into a lunge with your right leg, and, as you do, pass the kettlebell to your right hand; then position the bell toward the inside of your left leg (see Figure 10-11a).**

3. **Pass the kettlebell under your left leg so that your left hand can grab the bell as you push off with your left heel to stand up tall (see Figure 10-11b).**

4. **Step back into a lunge with your left leg, and, as you do, pass the kettlebell to your left hand; then position it toward the inside of your right leg.**

Keep your torso erect and tall as you step back into the lunge and pass the kettlebell under your leg.

5. **Pass the kettlebell under your right leg so that your right hand can grab the bell as you push off with your right heel to stand up tall.**

Continue to alternate sides for a total of 20 repetitions.

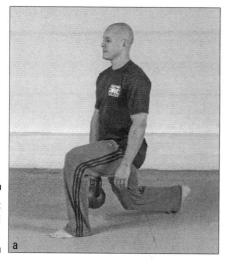 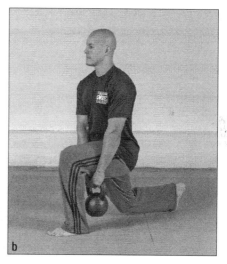

Figure 10-11: The tactical lunge.

a   b

If you have trouble passing the bell from one hand to the other as you're lunging, perform a traditional reverse lunge while holding the kettlebell by the horns with both hands (see Chapter 15 for details on how to do the reverse lunge). After you're steady and stable with the reverse lunge, you can pass the bell from one hand to the other.

The Deck Squat

I purposefully saved the *deck squat* for last in this chapter because it's a rather challenging exercise. In fact, in a class I was teaching, I called out, "Deck squats!" to cue students to the exercise, and one student innocently repeated, "Death squats?" In all honesty, deck squats won't kill you, but they aren't easy and you do need to have a lot of flexibility in your hips and strength in your glutes to do the exercise properly. In this section, I offer you some techniques that, with a little practice and patience, will get you doing the death squat — I mean deck squat — in no time.

Performing the basic deck squat

The deck squat is difficult because it requires that you get into a rock-bottom squat (see Chapter 8), then sit in a controlled motion to the floor, then roll back onto your back, and, finally, fire back up to a standing position without any hesitation. Sounds fun, right? It is fun; plus, the deck squat works your entire body, including your abs, increases your flexibility, and gets your heart rate up. After you've mastered the deck squat, you can create infinite combinations of equally intense exercises, like a deck squat with a jump squat, a deck squat with a press, a deck squat with a snatch, and so on and so forth.

To do the deck squat, use a floor that's matted or carpeted, and follow these steps:

1. **Stand with your feet shoulder width apart, and hold your kettlebell by the horns; your arms are in front of your body.**

2. **Reach back with your hips as if you're doing a rock-bottom front squat, and, as you approach the ground, slowly sit back onto your rear end (see Figure 10-12a).**

   Take care not to "fall" into this position for risk of hurting your tail bone. Sit down slowly.

3. **Roll back on your spine, letting your legs and feet follow you; keep the kettlebell at chest level (see Figure 10-12b).**

4. **Use your legs to give you some momentum and snap your hips to fire back up into the rock-bottom squat position, project the kettlebell straight out in front of you to act as a counterbalance; in one controlled motion, drive back up through your heels to stand in the position described in Step 1.**

   See Chapter 4 for more on how to snap your hips properly.

Perform ten repetitions.

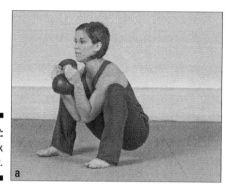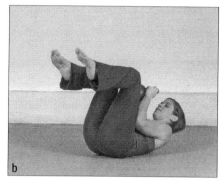

Figure 10-12:
The deck
squat.

Make sure to keep your hands on the kettlebell at all times. Don't use your hands for assistance, and don't cross your legs when coming up. Position your legs and feet shoulder width apart to drive up as you do in a front squat (see Chapter 8).

Using different methods to help you perform the deck squat successfully

If you're having trouble with the deck squat, you can try a couple of alternative methods that will eventually help you perform this exercise correctly:

✔ The box squat is the best alternative to the deck squat if you're having trouble getting into the rock-bottom squat position and getting back up with good form. I describe the box squat in detail in Chapter 6, but make sure you don't actually perform the roll-back portion of the deck squat exercise during the box squat. Also make sure the box you use during the box squat is no higher than 15 inches. Using the box to facilitate getting into rock-bottom position and then removing the box and practicing the actual deck squat trains your body how to properly do the exercise.

✔ If the box squat isn't a good option for you (because you don't own a plyometric box or because you want to perform the roll back portion of the deck squat exercise), use a BOSU as your target for the rock-bottom portion of the exercise. With the BOSU, you can perform the roll-back portion of the exercise *if* your abdominals are strong enough to stabilize you as you roll back. If your abs aren't strong enough and you end up rolling off the side of the BOSU (don't worry, only your pride will be hurt!), just practice the rock-bottom portion with the BOSU by tapping your butt to it before firing back up (as I describe in Step 4 in the preceding section). Then go back and practice the deck squat on the floor after you can perform the BOSU version with ease.

In addition, using the kettlebell as a counterbalance makes the deck squat easier. Try doing the deck squat without a kettlebell and see how much more difficult it is to get up!

My experience with students is not that they have a problem getting down and rolling back; they just can't get themselves up from the rock-bottom position. This problem generally indicates a lack of glute and leg strength. Practicing the rock-bottom squat in Chapter 8, in addition to using the alternatives listed in the preceding list, will help you do this exercise. If all else fails and you just can't do the deck squat, don't sweat it. You can do plenty of other lower-body exercises to strengthen and tone your lower half, such as swings (Chapter 6), squats (Chapter 8), single-leg dead lifts (earlier in this chapter), and tactical lunges (earlier in this chapter).

Chapter 11

Whittle Your Middle: Core Exercises

*P*eople tend to think the core consists only of the abdominal muscles; however, your core actually includes your whole trunk. Put simply, your core is everything but your arms and legs. A strong core makes all of life's movements seem effortless (which is the real reason why you should want a strong core — not for cosmetic appeal). On the other hand, a weak core not only makes everyday activities more difficult and strenuous but is also a recipe for injury. Your core should be the powerhouse of your body, but it can't be unless it's properly trained — which, as you may imagine, is where this chapter comes in.

The benefits of training your core with kettlebells include the following:

✔ A strong core makes performing everyday activities effortless.

✔ A strong core allows you to get better results from physical or sport-specific training programs.

✔ A strong core makes injuries less likely.

✔ A strong core makes for a sleek and sexy midsection.

✔ A strong core translates into a strong spine and strong connective tissues, which make physical exercise easier.

You don't find many practical strength-training programs (that is, programs the nonathlete can learn easily) that can match the core strength you gain from kettlebells. Olympic lifting comes close, but you can't swing a barbell between your legs, and chances are you won't have to clean and press 400 pounds to see the results you're looking for!

This chapter focuses on core-specific exercises that you can add to your regular kettlebell routine to help you obtain the power core that may have eluded you in other workout programs. You can do all the exercises in this chapter before, during, or after your regular routine.

You get the most benefit out of your core training when it involves full-body movements that tax a major portion of your body's musculature. Exercises like the swing (see Chapter 6), the clean (see Chapter 8), the military press (see Chapter 8), and the snatch (see Chapter 12) are perfect examples of full-body exercises that make your core stronger. So be sure to include these exercises in your routine along with the more core-specific exercises I describe in this chapter.

The Hot Potato

The *hot potato* exercise not only helps you master abdominal bracing and diaphragmatic breathing but also works your entire core (see Chapter 5 for complete instructions on bracing and breathing). It's important to use a challenging-enough size kettlebell to get the full benefits from the hot potato, but even if you were to use a very light kettlebell, you'd still experience a good core workout just from bracing and breathing throughout the exercise (see Chapter 3 for tips on selecting the right bell size). Put this exercise anywhere in your workout routine — before, during, or after your main workout — to work your core and to get in touch with your bracing and breathing power.

During the hot potato, make sure you use a matted or sturdy flooring surface, and clear your workout area of children and pets — just in case you drop your bell!

To do the hot potato, follow these steps:

1. **Stand with your feet slightly narrower than shoulder width apart, your abs braced for a punch, your glutes pinched, and your knees locked; have the bell part of the kettlebell in your left palm, handle facing downward, and your left elbow snug to your left side.**

2. **Put your right hand and arm in the same position as your left so that your right hand is ready to take the kettlebell when you pass it from your left hand; inhale (see Figure 11-1a).**

3. **As you forcefully exhale, pass the kettlebell from your left hand to your right, keeping your elbows snug to your sides, abs braced, and glutes pinched (see Figure 11-1b).**

Be sure to follow the kettlebell with your eyes throughout this movement.

Be careful not to pass the bell too close to your face; you certainly don't want to brush the kettlebell up against your face by accident!

4. **Inhale, then exhale forcefully as you pass the bell from your right hand to your left hand.**

Perform as many reps as you can while keeping good form for one minute. Work up to a steady and controlled pace, being mindful of your abs and glutes and breathing forcefully and with intention as you continue to pass the bell from hand to hand.

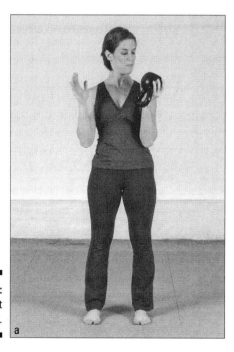
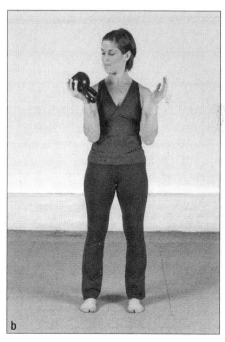

Figure 11-1:
The hot
potato.

a   b

Pretending that you're actually passing a hot potato from hand to hand helps you keep a steady pace.

Make sure to drive your heels through the ground, keep your abs, glutes, and thighs tight, and maintain a tall spine throughout the movement. Your body should be a solid column while performing the hot potato.

The Seated Russian Twist

The _Seated Russian twist_ is a core exercise that specifically targets your oblique muscles; you can perform it before, during, or after your workout. Like with the hot potato exercise in the preceding section, as long as you're bracing and breathing properly throughout the movement, you'll feel it in your core.

For the seated Russian twist, you can experiment with a kettlebell that's one size lighter than the one you use for swings (see Chapter 6); if you have only one kettlebell available, use it and adjust the number of reps as needed. The seated Russian twist can also be done effectively without a kettlebell; to do so, go through the following steps, pretending to hold an imaginary kettlebell.

To do the seated Russian twist, follow these steps:

1. **Sit on the floor, holding your kettlebell by the horns at your chest; bend your knees and keep them together, bring your heels off the floor, squeeze your glutes and abs, and inhale (see Figure 11-2a).**

    To hold the bell by the horns, position two hands on either side of the middle of the handle.

2. **Twist your torso to the left side and let your eyes follow the movement so that you're looking to the left as you twist (see Figure 11-2b).**

    As you twist, keep holding the kettlebell by the horns with your elbows close to your rib cage; keep the kettlebell close to your chest and forcefully exhale with each twist.

3. **Return to the center position in Step 1; then twist to the right side.**

Continue to alternate sides, and perform as many reps as you can with good form in 30 seconds.

Many people with a weak core move more from the hips than from the torso while performing the seated Russian twist. Make sure your movement originates from your torso and not your hips. To keep your body aware of where you're moving from, place a sneaker or small medicine ball between your knees and squeeze it throughout the movement. This method has the added benefit of giving your abdominal muscles even more of a workout.

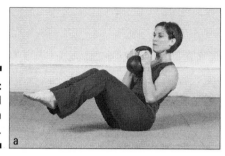 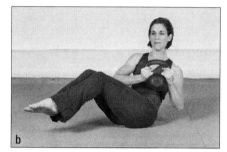

Figure 11-2: The seated Russian twist.

Don't worry if you need to have your heels on the floor when you first perform the seated Russian twist; just try to work up to bringing your heels off the ground for maximum benefit.

Ready for a challenge? Straighten your arms, and hold the kettlebell at arms' distance in front of you while twisting from side to side. Keep your shoulders down and away from your ears, and make sure to engage your lat muscles during the movement.

The Renegade Row with Two Kettlebells

The *renegade row with two kettlebells* is a highly effective core exercise that challenges your muscles to work in unison to perform the exercise properly. You need two kettlebells of the same size to perform this version of the renegade row — don't worry, the exercise is well worth the investment of buying another kettlebell! (Check out the one-bell version of the renegade row in Chapter 10.)

Note that you need to use two kettlebells that are at least 26 pounds each for the two-bell renegade row. Smaller kettlebells can't support and stabilize your weight and are unsafe to use with this exercise.

The renegade row with two kettlebells is a difficult exercise to master. In fact, the first time I did this exercise in the gym with dumbbells (which is a little different from how you do it with kettlebells), I almost did a face plant. Be prepared to fall to one side the first few times you attempt this version of the renegade row, and make sure you practice this exercise on a level and soft surface (firm matting that absorbs your fall is best).

To do the renegade row with two kettlebells, follow these steps:

1. **Begin in a plank or push-up position with your kettlebells shoulder width apart, your hands positioned on the kettlebell handles, your shoulders positioned directly over your hands, your hips square, and your arms straightened (see Figure 11-3a).**

   Keep your eye gaze down toward the floor throughout this exercise.

2. **Tighten your abs, glutes, and thighs; with your left hand, lift the kettlebell off the ground and row it toward your left hip as you push your right hand straight down onto the handle of your right kettlebell to stabilize you (see Figure 11-3b).**

   Your right hand remains steady on the other kettlebell, acting as a support for your body.

3. **Slowly and in a controlled motion, return the left kettlebell to the ground to the start position I describe in Step 1.**

   Keep your hips square throughout the movement.

   Visualize placing the kettlebell on a glass table every time you return it to the ground. Doing so helps you maintain control throughout the exercise.

4. **Repeat Steps 2 and 3 for your right side.**

Continue to alternate sides, and perform a total of ten repetitions (one rep consists of a row on each side).

Keep your shoulders over the handles of the bells during the renegade row. If you reach too far out for the kettlebells during the exercise, you'll fall. Also, keep your wrists solid and locked while performing the exercise. Any break in the wrists will cause you to fall to one side or the other.

Figure 11-3:
The renegade row with two kettlebells.

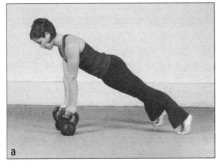
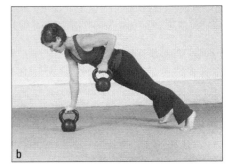

a

b

Putting It All Together: A 15-Minute Core Circuit

You can use the following core circuit either as a stand-alone program or as an addition before or after your regular kettlebell workout. You can go through it once a week or as many as three times a week. To do the circuit, go through each exercise without taking a break in between. You can rest for 30 to 45 seconds at the end of each round. Try to complete 2 rounds in 15 minutes.

- ✔ Exercise 1: Hot potato for 1 minute
- ✔ Exercise 2: Seated Russian twist for 1 minute
- ✔ Exercise 3: Hot potato for 1 minute
- ✔ Exercise 4: Renegade row with two kettlebells (20 total reps)
- ✔ Exercise 5: Seated Russian twist for 1 minute
- ✔ Exercise 6: Hot potato for 1 minute
- ✔ Exercise 7: Renegade row with two kettlebells (20 total reps)

Chapter 12

Mastering the Five Ultimate Kettlebell Exercises

Typically, students at my gym, Iron Core, are ready to progress to more advanced kettlebell exercises after they thoroughly master the basics. Because every individual comes to the gym with different fitness and skill levels, there's no set time when this progression happens. But everyone — no matter the fitness level — follows a certain progression; for example, after people master the clean and press (see Chapter 8), they move on to the clean and jerk. After they're able to perform all the swing variations I describe in Chapter 6 and can clean and press the bell well, they move on to the snatch.

If you've fully mastered the techniques in Chapters 4 and 5 and the basic exercises in Part II, you're probably ready to try out the exercises in this chapter. (You have an even better chance of succeeding with these exercise if you can do the exercises in Chapters 10 and 11, too.) However, the exercises in this chapter are more advanced, and some of them may prove quite difficult to master simply because you don't have the skills you need initially. But don't worry — skills can be learned and then honed, and, with patience and discipline, you can master these exercises as well as you mastered those in the previous chapters. For all the exercises in this chapter, I offer suggestions and variations that can help you in your quest for a strong and lean body.

Mastering the clean and jerk and the snatch are well worth the time and frustration they may take because they really pump up your strength and endurance. The overhead squat, Sots press, and pistol exercises are at the advanced end of the kettlebell spectrum; even if you can't master these exercises, rest assured that you have more than enough tools in your box to continue progressing with kettlebells. But why not give them a try?

The Clean and Jerk

After you master the clean and press in Chapter 8, you can move on to the *clean and jerk* with confidence. This advanced exercise is a variation of the clean and press that engages your body from head to toe and tests your muscle and cardiovascular endurance.

To do the clean and jerk, follow these steps:

1. **Stand with your feet about shoulder width apart and your glutes and abs tightened.**

2. **Clean the kettlebell to the rack on your left side, keeping your elbow close to your rib cage (see Figure 12-1a).**

   To clean the bell to the rack, turn your kettlebell so it's facing sideways, sit back into your hips, place your left hand on the kettlebell handle with your thumb pointing backward, and aggressively snap your hips to bring the kettlebell to the rack. Flip to Chapter 8 for all the details on how to clean the kettlebell.

3. **To begin the jerk portion of the exercise, push your hips slightly back and bend your knees slightly (see Figure 12-1b).**

4. **Begin to straighten up your body very quickly to "bump" the kettlebell from your chest (see Figure 12-1c); without any hesitation continue with Step 5.**

   Make sure you use your hips to move the bell initially.

5. **Get under the kettlebell and absorb the weight by pushing your hips back, bending your knees again, and straightening your left arm into the locked-out position (see Figure 12-1d); drive through your heels with a forceful stomp to stand up tall (see Figure 12-1e).**

   Make sure to keep your shoulders in their sockets, and tighten your lats, thighs, glutes, and abs at the top of the movement. Your left arm is in a fully locked-out overhead position at the top of the movement; your right arm is down at your side throughout the exercise.

   Think *push hips back, bump, absorb, get tall,* all in one fluid motion when performing the jerk portion of the clean and jerk.

6. **From the top overhead locked-out position, let the bell descend back into the rack position by bending your knees and bracing your abs to absorb the weight of the bell coming into the rack position. After the bell is in the rack position, stand back up tall and re-clean the kettlebell to the start position I describe in Steps 1 and 2.**

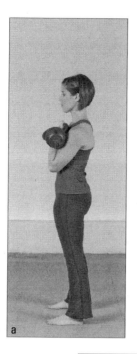
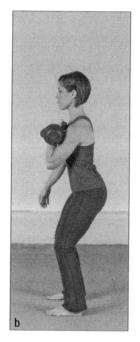
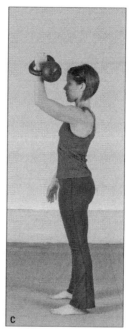
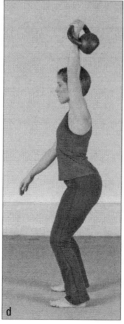
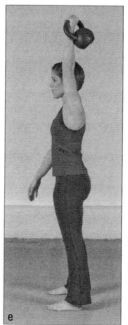

Figure 12-1:
The clean
and jerk.

Getting the scoop on Girevoy Sport

The clean and jerk and the snatch are two exercises that rev up your workout significantly by increasing both your strength and endurance. You can even find competitions for both of these exercises that test competitors' stamina. Called *Girevoy Sport*, or *GS*, these competitions push athletes to the ultimate limit as they try to perform as many repetitions of each exercise as they can within a ten-minute time frame without setting down the kettlebell. Winners become Master of Sport. Many years ago, I competed in GS and became a Candidate Master of Sport (the female designation). Find out more about GS at www. usgsf.com or www.girevoysport.ru.

Perform eight repetitions on the left side; switch sides by taking an extra swing (Chapter 6 has details on the alternating swing) or by setting down the kettlebell and re-cleaning it. Perform eight repetitions on the right side.

After you practice all your repetitions, try performing the exercise for one minute — 30 seconds on each side. If you aren't out of breath after doing so, you need a heavier bell. In fact, the exercise lends itself to using a heavier weight overhead than you normally would be able to press. Why? You don't just engage your lower body to help you move through this exercise; the second dip described in Step 5 (when you push back into your hips and bend your knees for the second time) allows your whole body to absorb the impact of a heavier bell.

If you succeed at doing the clean and jerk, try doing this exercise with two kettlebells of the same size. Follow the steps for the one-kettlebell clean and jerk, but clean and jerk both bells at the same time. See if you can work for up to ten minutes without setting down the kettlebells. You can "rest" in the rack if need be.

The Snatch

The *snatch* is one of the most dynamic full-body kettlebell exercises out there — it takes your strength, flexibility, endurance, and power to entirely new levels. Being able to snatch well allows your body to fully understand how to generate force and power, which carries over nicely into your life and sport-specific activities. Although the basics of the exercise (taught here in Girevoy Sport style) aren't hard to learn after you understand the hip snap that I describe in Chapter 4, the many nuances in the exercise will take time and practice to master.

Note: You should be able to snatch the same size kettlebell that you're able to press with control and precision and that you're comfortable using for the one-arm swing that I describe in Chapter 6.

To help you get started with the snatch, practice the high pull from Chapter 10, the one-arm swing from Chapter 6, and the press from Chapter 8. The snatch incorporates these exercises in one fluid motion, so knowing how to do each exercise separately will help you master the snatch more easily.

To do the snatch, follow these steps:

1. **Stand with your feet slightly wider than shoulder width apart with the kettlebell on the ground between your feet with the handle positioned sideways.**

2. **Push your hips back to reach down for your bell with your left hand, thumb pointing back.**

3. **Use a backswing to get the kettlebell off the ground, snap your hips, and drive your heels through the ground as you bring the kettlebell up in front of your body, with your left elbow bent (see Figure 12-2a); punch up and through the bell in one fluid motion to get the bell into the top position over your head (see Figure 12-2b).**

   Tame the arc of the kettlebell by imagining you're zipping up your jacket; aggressively punch the bell up as it approaches your chest. Don't hesitate at the shoulder like you do in the clean and press.

   At the top position, your left arm is fully extended and locked out, and your wrist is solid and not broken or bent. Be sure to pinch your glutes, thighs, and abs at the top, as well, taking care not to let the kettlebell throw you back; keep your heels pressed into the ground, your body solid as a column, and your shoulder connected to the lat muscle.

   At the top of the exercise, the kettlebell handle should rest from the web of your thumb to the outer part of your palm and wrist, not straight across your palm (refer to Figure 12-2b). Ensure this positioning by turning your thumb back at the backswing of the movement.

4. **Bring your kettlebell down by corkscrewing the bell down in front of you in one fluid motion; push your hips back as your bring the bell into the backswing position.**

   To corkscrew the bell, simply rotate your hand as you bring the bell down so that your pinky faces inward at about chest height until you push back into your hips at the bottom of the exercise and begin to point your thumb backward to get into the position described in Step 2.

Perform five repetitions on the left side by repeating Steps 3 and 4; use an extra swing to switch sides (see Chapter 6 for details on the alternating swing), and perform five repetitions on the right.

The snatch is one fluid, dynamic movement. You aren't pressing the bell up; rather, you're using the force generated from your hips to get the bell into the top position. Your hips do all the work — your arm is simply the guide.

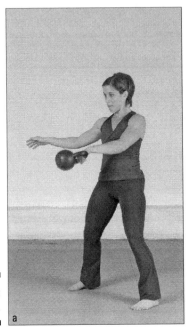 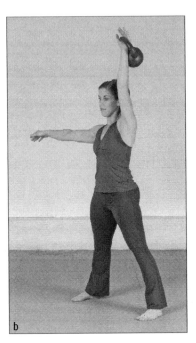

Figure 12-2:
The snatch.

a   b

You shouldn't feel the kettlebell bang or slap your wrist when performing the snatch. If you're banging your wrist at the top of the movement, you may not be keeping a bend in your elbow as you make your way up to the top position; or, you may not be generating enough force from your hips for the kettlebell to simply float up into the top position.

If you're slapping your wrist at the top, practice the high pull from Chapter 10 to help you correct your form. In addition, practice a bent-arm, one-arm swing. To do so, follow the instructions for the one-arm swing in Chapter 6, but have a slight bend in your arm as you bring the kettlebell to the top position (at chest height). Make sure the swing is at least shoulder height so that each one of the swings could turn into a snatch if you were to punch through to bring the bell to the top position.

The RKC style is a more hard-style form that doesn't incorporate the corkscrew method on the descent of the exercise. Just make sure it still feels and looks smooth at the top, with no banging of the wrist.

The Overhead Squat

If you can reach a rock-bottom squat and perform a military press with full lockout (see Chapter 8 for details on both moves), you're already halfway to mastering the *overhead squat,* another high-intensity kettlebell exercise. Now you just have to master the other half. In this section, I outline how to do the overhead squat and give you several techniques for correcting your form.

If you find that you just can't perform the overhead squat, don't worry. Very few people I've taught can do the exercise properly; even so, they've been able to radically change their overall strength, flexibility, and body composition just by working toward it. So, if you can do a rock-bottom squat and achieve full lockout in the military press, at least give this exercise a try.

The basic overhead squat

When you begin to work on the overhead squat, use a kettlebell that's one size lighter than the one you use for swings or one that's the size you can confidently use for the Turkish get-up. If you have trouble with the overhead squat, refer to the corrective exercises I describe in the next section.

To do the overhead squat, follow these steps.

1. **Stand with your feet about shoulder width apart and your glutes and abs tightened.**

2. **Clean the kettlebell to the rack on your left side.**

   Check out Chapter 8 if you need a refresher on cleaning.

3. **Press the bell up into full lockout position.**

   As you press the bell up, your left arm is locked out overhead, with your shoulders in their sockets and your lats tight; your right arm is at your side. See Chapter 8 for more details on pressing the kettlebell.

4. **Keep your eyes on the kettlebell, slowly sit back into your hips, with your weight on your heels, and pull yourself down into a rock-bottom squat, all the while keeping the kettlebell steady and controlled in the lockout position (see Figure 12-3).**

5. **After you reach rock-bottom position, drive up through your heels and stand up tall, keeping your abs and glutes pinched and your left arm locked out.**

   Don't let your left arm or kettlebell drift forward or let the elbow break during this movement.

Perform five repetitions on the left side while keeping the kettlebell in the full lockout position (don't bring it into the rack until all reps are complete). Then switch sides by bringing the kettlebell back down into the rack, taking an extra swing to switch sides (see Chapter 6 for details on the alternating swing), or setting down the kettlebell and re-cleaning it on the right side. Perform five repetitions on the right side.

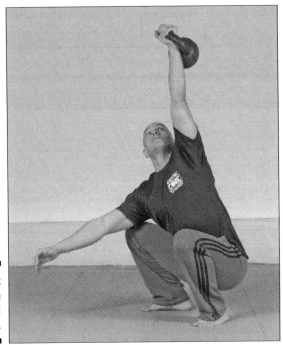

Figure 12-3: The overhead squat.

Corrective drills for the overhead squat

If your form during the overhead squat is less than ideal, take a look at the corrective drills I describe in this section. They can help you fix your form so you get the maximum benefit from this exercise.

In addition to the techniques I describe in this section, two other kettlebell exercises can help you make progress with the overhead squat:

✔ **Overhead squat Turkish get-up:** Many of my students can perform the overhead squat version of the Turkish get-up (see Chapter 7) but struggle with the basic overhead squat. When I point out to them that they're actually doing an overhead squat already, they have more confidence in themselves and their abilities and go on to master the overhead squat.

✔ **Deck squat:** This exercise helps you practice getting into rock-bottom position and getting back up to a standing position from the ground (see Chapter 10).

The barbell or broomstick overhead squat

If you find that your arm drifts forward or your elbow breaks during the overhead squat or that you just can't get into the rock-bottom squat position, you can use the *barbell overhead squat* to help fix your form. If you don't have a barbell, use a broomstick. The idea behind this corrective technique is to get your body moving in the right pattern; using less weight can help you focus on your form rather than your strength.

To do this version of the overhead squat, follow the steps from the section "The basic overhead squat," but instead of holding a kettlebell in one hand, hold a barbell or broomstick in a wide grip with both hands. Perform ten total repetitions without setting down the barbell or broomstick.

Practice this variation of the overhead squat until you feel ready to go back and attempt the kettlebell version of the exercise.

The overhead squat with a target

Having a target, such as a plyometric box or a BOSU, to reach for helps some people perform the overhead squat, especially when they lack the body awareness to know how low they're getting or aren't getting in the rock-bottom position. If you own either of these pieces of equipment (preferably one that's 8 to 12 inches tall), do the target version of the overhead squat by following the steps described in the section "The basic overhead squat," using the box or BOSU as your guide for the squatting movement. Practice this drill with your kettlebell.

Make sure you stand far enough away from the target that you're still able to push back into your hips when initiating the squatting movement, but not too far away that you miss the box when squatting down. Also make sure you don't put your weight on the box or BOSU; instead, just tap the box lightly with your rear end and drive up to the top standing position.

Avoiding caved-in knees and raised heels with the band squat

You may be able to perform the rock-bottom squat, but, if your knees cave inward or your heels come off the floor when you're loading your body from the overhead position, you likely have an imbalance in your form. Use the band squat corrective technique from Chapter 8 to clean up your form.

The Sots Press

After you master the rock-bottom squat from Chapter 8, you should be comfortable enough in the rock-bottom position that you can stay in it for 30 seconds or more (without kettlebells). If you can do so, take some time to try the *Sots press,* which is a great combination of squat and press that challenges your strength, flexibility, and balance. It's a fun exercise to do and can serve as a challenging alternative to the military press that I describe in Chapter 8.

To do the Sots press, follow these steps:

1. **Stand with your feet about shoulder width apart and your glutes and abs tightened.**

2. **Clean the kettlebell to the rack on your left side.**

   If you need a refresher on cleaning, flip to Chapter 8.

3. **Get into the rock-bottom front squat by pushing your hips back and letting your knees follow your lead as you descend (see Figure 12-4a).**

   See Chapter 8 for instructions on doing the rock-bottom front squat.

   After you get in the rock-bottom position, your heels can be on or off the floor for the Sots press. In either case, make sure the weight is distributed evenly between your left and right sides.

4. **Letting your eyes follow the kettlebell, press the bell up from the rack position into the full lockout overhead position of the military press (see Figure 12-4b).**

   Your left bicep should be in line with your left ear in the lockout position.

5. **Return the kettlebell to the rack position on the left side while maintaining the rock-bottom squat position.**

Perform five repetitions on the left side by repeating Steps 4 and 5. Switch sides by setting down the kettlebell and standing back up to re-clean the kettlebell on the right side; perform five repetitions on the right side.

Don't let your knees cave inward or let your knees come past your toes during the Sots press exercise. Both errors in form will cause knee pain. To correct bad form, use the band squat or barbell or broomstick squat I describe in the section "Corrective drills for the overhead squat."

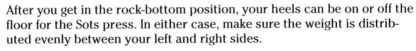

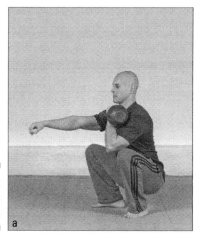 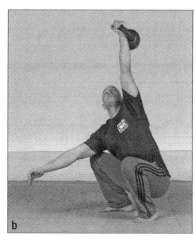

Figure 12-4:
The Sots
press.

The Pistol: The Ultimate in Leg and Glute Strength

The *pistol* is the ultimate exercise for building and maintaining leg and glute strength. It requires you to have a good amount of hamstring and glute flexibility and hip mobility. Indeed, you perform a feat of strength every time you do one the right way.

Before you get started with the pistol, be aware — pistols are difficult to perform. To help you achieve success with pistols, I offer several variations in the following sections; you can perform pistols with just your body weight or with one kettlebell. I also explain how to correct poor pistol form.

The pistol without a kettlebell

Don't think that this version of the pistol is a piece of cake to perform just because it doesn't use a kettlebell. Indeed, it's quite challenging — not to mention effective. Be sure you practice the pistol without the kettlebell before trying the weighted version because, if you attempt to do the pistol with a kettlebell without making sure you have the flexibility and strength to do so, you'll most likely fall on your butt! In all my years of teaching this exercise, I've encountered only one person who could perform the pistol with a kettlebell immediately — my younger brother, who's strong and flexible and who was naïve enough to believe he could do it.

To do the pistol without a kettlebell, follow these steps:

1. **Stand with your feet together, and then lift your left leg off the ground and straighten it out in front of you; bring your arms out in front of you and tighten your abs (see Figure 12-5a).**

2. **Slowly sit back into your hips until your right glute is touching your right calf muscle in the rock-bottom position (see Figure 12-5b).**

   Keep your right heel on the ground and abs tight throughout the movement.

3. **Drive through your right heel, activating your hamstrings, glutes, and abs, to stand up tall without using your arms or other leg for assistance.**

   Don't bounce in the bottom of the movement; instead, aggressively push through the right heel to get up.

Perform three reps on the right leg and three reps on the left leg.

The pistol without a kettlebell can actually be more challenging than performing the exercise with a bell, so use a small counterweight like a medicine ball to help you keep your balance while you learn the exercise. You can also position your arms out at your sides and pretend to push two walls away as you push through your heel to come up to standing.

Don't let your heel come off the ground during the exercise, and don't let your torso fall forward. Both errors in form could cause injury. Practice the assisted-pistol corrective drill I describe in the section "Fixing form with the assisted pistol" if you're making either of these form mistakes.

The pistol with a kettlebell

To perform the pistol with a kettlebell, you can hold the bell either by the horns (by grabbing either side of the middle of the handle with both hands and holding it at about chest height) or in the rack position (see Chapter 8 for rack-position basics). For beginners, I recommend holding it by the horns because it can act as a counterweight to assist you in getting up out of the rock-bottom position. Also, as you begin practicing the pistol, try to use a kettlebell that's one or two sizes lighter than the kettlebell you use for swings.

To do the pistol while holding the kettlebell by the horns, follow the steps for the nonweighted pistol in the preceding section, but this time, hold your kettlebell by the horns (see Figure 12-6). Perform three repetitions on each side.

To perform the pistol while holding the kettlebell in the rack position, follow the steps for the nonweighted pistol in the preceding section, but this time, start by cleaning the kettlebell into the rack position (refer to Chapter 8 for more on cleaning the kettlebell).

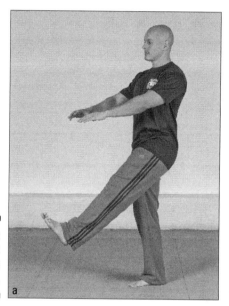
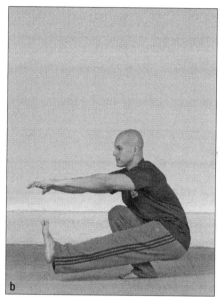

Figure 12-5:
The pistol without a kettlebell.

a

b

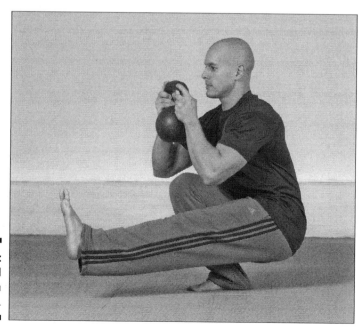

Figure 12-6:
The pistol with a kettlebell.

Fixing form with the assisted pistol

For this corrective drill, you need a sturdy exercise band that has minimal stretch or a yoga strap, along with a pull-up bar, column, or solid door with a doorknob. Take your band or strap and position it around the pull-up bar to act as a device to help you keep your form throughout the movement and to assist you in getting up from rock-bottom position.

To do the assisted pistol, follow the instructions for the nonweighted pistol that I describe in the section "The pistol without a kettlebell," this time using your pull-up bar and strap to assist you (see Figure 12-7); perform five repetitions on the right leg and five repetitions on the left leg.

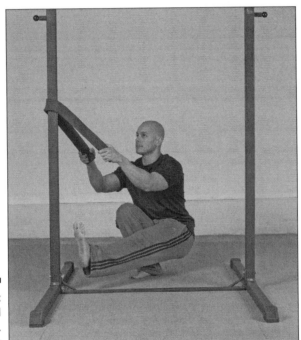

Figure 12-7:
The assisted
pistol.

Keep in mind the following pointers as you perform the assisted-pistol corrective drill:

✓ **Don't rely on the band too much when pulling yourself up.** Use the band to assist you in getting up, but don't struggle so much with the band that you feel like you're going to break apart the pull-up bar when you come up!

✔ **Keep your working heel on the ground throughout the exercise.** If you can't keep your heel down, chances are you lack the flexibility to do so, which means you need to do some exercises that increase your mobility in the hamstrings and glutes before you can perform the pistol properly. Some good exercises to try are the swing (Chapter 6), the windmill (Chapter 11), and the single-leg dead lift (Chapter 10).

Building Endurance and Strength with Five Fiery Five-Minute Workouts

The following workouts are short and intense and meant to serve as practice sets, but they also build endurance and strength. You can try out these exercises on the days when you want a break from your regular kettlebell routine or use them to warm up for your light-day workouts. The combinations are meant to be performed on different days, so don't do any more than one of the workouts on any given day.

If you want to do these short, intense workouts before your regular routine, good complementary exercises include the following:

✔ Swing variations (see Chapter 6)

✔ The Turkish get-up (see Chapter 7)

✔ Squat variations (see Chapter 8)

✔ The windmill (see Chapter 10)

✔ Lunge variations (like the tactical lunge in Chapter 10)

✔ Row variations (see Chapters 10 and 11)

✔ Body weight exercises such as pull-ups and push-ups

Warm up for about two or three minutes for the following workouts using your choice of warm-up options from Chapter 5. All the workouts are for time, so you need to have a good stopwatch or Gymboss handy. Start your timer as soon as you're ready to begin your first exercise (don't time your warm-up), set it for five minutes, and try to move through the circuit without stopping.

Workout 1: Leg- and glute-endurance builder

If you're interested in building leg and glute endurance, this five-minute blast will certainly do the job. Both exercises in this workout really tax your lower body and give your heart rate a big jump.

- ✔ Exercise 1: Pistol (three reps on each side)

- ✔ Exercise 2: Clean and jerk for 30 seconds on each side with no rest in between sides (one minute total)

- ✔ Exercise 3: Pistol (two reps on each side)

- ✔ Exercise 4: Clean and jerk for 30 seconds on each side with no rest in between sides (one minute total)

- ✔ Exercise 5: Pistol (one rep on each side)

- ✔ Exercise 6: Clean and jerk for 20 seconds on each side with no rest in between sides (40 seconds total)

Workout 2: Upper-body strengthener and cardio-endurance builder

Because both the snatch and the overhead squat require you to bring the kettlebell overhead, the following workout taxes your upper body considerably. The overhead squat also gives your glutes and legs a workout, and both exercises test your cardiovascular endurance.

- ✔ Exercise 1: Snatch for 30 seconds on each side with no rest in between sides (one minute total)

- ✔ Exercise 2: Overhead squat (five reps on each side)

- ✔ Exercise 3: Snatch for 30 seconds on each side with no rest in between sides (one minute total)

- ✔ Exercise 4: Overhead squat (five reps on each side)

- ✔ Exercise 5: Snatch for 30 seconds on each side with no rest in between sides (one minute total)

Workout 3: Upper- and lower-body strengthener

If you want to blast your upper and lower body and get your heart rate up at the same time, the following five-minute workout is perfect for you. When you're performing the Sots press in this workout, your legs will probably start to feel fatigued from the pistols, but that's part of the fun, right?

✔ Exercise 1: Pistol (four reps on each side)

✔ Exercise 2: Sots press (five reps on each side)

✔ Exercise 3: Pistol (three reps on each side)

✔ Exercise 4: Sots press (five reps on each side)

✔ Exercise 5: Pistol (two reps on each side)

✔ Exercise 6: Sots press (five reps on each side)

Workout 4: Lower-body strengthener and cardio-endurance builder

The clean and jerk is a great lower-body-endurance builder, but it also gives you an intense cardiovascular workout. During this workout, do the following:

✔ Perform the clean and jerk for 30 seconds on each side (one minute total).

✔ Rest for 20 seconds.

Repeat this circuit for five minutes, resting 20 seconds in between each clean and jerk set. Try to complete four full circuits.

Workout 5: Cardio-endurance builder and fat burner

Being able to snatch for five minutes with minimal or no rest is a rite of passage in the world of kettlebells, so use this workout to build up your cardiovascular endurance and perfect your snatch form. Not surprisingly, this workout is excellent for fat burning, too.

During this workout, do the following:

✔ Perform the snatch for 30 seconds on each side (one minute total).

✔ Rest for 20 seconds.

Repeat this circuit for five minutes, resting 20 seconds in between each snatch set. Try to complete four full circuits.

Chapter 13

Kicking It Up a Notch with Advanced Kettlebell Workouts and Combinations

....

In This Chapter

▶ Burning fat and increasing power and strength

▶ Trying some great kettlebell combinations

▶ Adding even more variety with combo workouts

....

*J*ust as the beginner workouts in Chapter 9 guide your first four weeks to a leaner and stronger new you, the workouts and combos in this chapter take you through your next four to six weeks to help you make even more progress. At this point in your workouts, you may need to bump up the weight of your kettlebell or just mix up your routine so you continue to be challenged and get results. After you've mastered the basics covered in Part II and made your way through the advanced moves in Chapters 10 through 12, you're ready to take your kettlebell workout to the next level. This chapter shows you how to put all those exercises together into cohesive and advanced workouts.

Each workout in this chapter is designed to last 25 to 30 minutes. Use one kettlebell for the workouts, and make sure to have a good stopwatch handy to time the exercises and rest breaks. (If you're using a kettlebell size that's challenging enough, you should need the rest period for *at least* the time indicated in the workouts; see Chapter 3 for more on choosing the right size kettlebell.)

I offer two-kettlebell options for each exercise in which you can use two kettlebells of the same size to get an even more intense workout. If you use two kettlebells, your skill level *must* be high — especially for two-kettlebell snatches.

Use the guidelines I lay out in Chapter 9 to decide how many days a week to work out and how to split up your workout days. Ideally, you'll engage in your kettlebell workouts two to four days a week.

Want even more variety in your routine? This chapter also offers you some popular kettlebell combination exercises, which I put into some fun combo workouts. Get ready to really get moving!

Advanced Workout 1: Flab to Fab

This workout includes three extremely dynamic exercises — the snatch, the swing, and a killer deck squat/snatch combination — that will leave you breathless after your first round. It also includes front squats, which tax your muscular endurance even more than usual because your legs are already tired from the other exercises in the workout. You burn tons of calories with this workout, so it's perfect for turning flab to fab in no time!

To warm up for this workout, do two or three dynamic stretches from Chapter 5 and two full Turkish get-up/high windmill combinations on each side (I describe this combination later in the section "Great Kettlebell Combinations to Try"). After your warm-up, perform the exercises listed in Table 13-1 to get going with the flab-to-fab workout.

Table 13-1	Advanced Flab-to Fab Workout				
Exercise	**Number of Reps or Time in Each Set**	**Number of Sets**	**Rest Period between Sets**	**Two-Kettlebell Option (Optional)**	**Reference Chapter**
Halo	1 minute	2	10 seconds	---	5
Snatch on the left	30 seconds	1	---	30 seconds	12
Snatch on the right	30 seconds	1	30 seconds after completing snatch on both sides	---	12
Two-arm swing	30 seconds	1	30 seconds	---	6
Front squat with kettlebell racked on the left	30 seconds	1	---	30 seconds	8

Exercise	Number of Reps or Time in Each Set	Number of Sets	Rest Period between Sets	Two-Kettlebell Option (Optional)	Reference Chapter
Front squat with kettle-bell racked on the right	30 seconds	1	30 seconds after com-pleting front squat on both sides	-----	8
Snatch on the left	30 seconds	1	---	30 seconds	12
Snatch on the right	30 seconds	1	30 seconds after complet-ing snatch on both sides	----	12
Deck squat	10 reps	1	30 seconds	---	10
Deck squat/ snatch combo on the left	30 seconds	1	---	---	13 (see the instruc-tions later in the sec-tion "Great Kettlebell Combinations to Try")
Deck squat/ snatch combo on the right	30 seconds	1	30 seconds after complet-ing combo on both sides	----	13 (see the instruc-tions later in the sec-tion "Great Kettlebell Combinations to Try")
Renegade row with two kettlebells	20 reps	2	30 seconds	---	11

To snatch two kettlebells at the same time, you need to be highly proficient with the one-arm snatch first. If you are, use the same technique you use to snatch one kettlebell, except snatch two bells at the same time. Your legs may need to be slightly wider apart, but all the other steps from Chapter 12 for the one-kettlebell version apply to the two-kettlebell version.

To perform the front squat with two kettlebells, rack one kettlebell on your left side and one on your right. Other than using two kettlebells, you go through all the same steps I describe for the one-kettlebell front squat in Chapter 8.

After you finish all the moves in Table 13-1, cool down with any three cool-down stretches or Z-Health movements from Chapter 5.

Advanced Workout 2: Cardio Burn

The combinations and dynamic exercises included in this workout and the few rest breaks you get to take make this workout a true cardio burn. The sets of swings that appear throughout the workout really make your heart work and increase your cardiovascular endurance.

To warm up for this workout, do two or three dynamic stretches from Chapter 5 and three high windmills on each side (see Chapter 10 for instructions). After you warm up, perform the exercises listed in Table 13-2 for your workout.

Table 13-2		Advanced Cardio-Burn Workout			
Exercise	*Number of Reps in Each Set*	*Number of Sets*	*Rest Period between Sets*	*Two-Kettlebell Option (Optional)*	*Reference Chapter*
Clean/squat combo on the right	10	1	---	20 reps	9 (for the combo); 8 (for individual moves)
Alternating swing	20	1	---	---	6
Clean/squat combo on the left	10	1	---	20 reps	9 (for the combo); 8 (for individual moves)
Alternating swing	20	1	30 seconds	---	6

Exercise	Number of Reps in Each Set	Number of Sets	Rest Period between Sets	Two-Kettlebell Option (Optional)	Reference Chapter
Snatch on the right	10	1	---	10 reps	12
Alternating swing	20	1	---	---	6
Snatch on the left	10	1	---	10 reps	12
Alternating swing	20	1	30 seconds	---	6
High pull on the right	10	1	---	---	10
Alternating swing	20	1	---	---	6
High pull on the left	10	1	---	---	10
Alternating swing	20	1	30 seconds	---	6
Clean and press on the right	10	1	---	20 reps	8
Alternating swing	20	1	---	---	6
Clean and press on the left	10	1	---	20 reps	8
Alternating swing	20	1	30 seconds	---	6
One-arm row on the right	10	1	---	Renegade row with two kettlebells	10; 11
Alternating swing	20	1	---	---	6
One-arm row on the left	10	1	---	Renegade row with two kettlebells	10; 11
Alternating swing	20	1	30 seconds	---	6

To perform the clean/squat combo with two kettlebells, clean both kettlebells into the rack at the same time, hold the bells in the rack for the squat portion of the combo, and re-clean the kettlebells to begin your next repetition.

All done? Cool down with any three cool-down stretches or Z-Health movements from Chapter 5.

Advanced Workout 3: Power and Strength

Like the beginner power-and-strength workout in Chapter 9, this advanced version uses lower reps, more sets, and more rest than a traditional kettlebell workout, which makes for an ideal opportunity to increase the size kettlebell you're using. This type of workout helps you gain power and strength and allows you to feel like you can really go the distance in your fat-burning and cardio-intensive workouts.

To warm up for this workout, do two or three stretches from Chapter 5 and four two-kettlebell windmills on each side (see Chapter 10 for instructions). After you warm up, perform the exercises listed in Table 13-3 for your workout.

To complete the power-and-strength workout, you can move through each exercise either by doing the repetitions and sets indicated and then moving to the next exercise or by performing one set of each exercise and then going back to the first exercise until you've completed all the sets.

Table 13-3	Advanced Power-and-Strength Workout				
Exercise	**Number of Reps in Each Set**	**Number of Sets**	**Rest Period between Sets**	**Two-Kettlebell Option (Optional)**	**Reference Chapter**
Clean and press on the left	5	4	---	25 to 30 seconds	8
Clean and press on the right	5	4	45 seconds after completing combo on both sides	---	8

Exercise	Number of Reps in Each Set	Number of Sets	Rest Period between Sets	Two-Kettlebell Option (Optional)	Reference Chapter
Single-leg dead lift on the left	5	4	---	---	10
Single-leg dead lift on the right	5	4	30 seconds after completing dead lift on both sides	---	10
Front squat on the left	5	4	---	30 seconds	8
Front squat on the right	5	4	30 seconds after completing squat on both sides	---	8
Renegade row with two kettlebells	20	4	30 seconds	---	11

When you're finished working out, cool down with any three cool-down stretches or Z-Health movements from Chapter 5.

Advanced Workout 4: Tabata Protocol

Designed to increase your muscular and cardiovascular endurance, *Tabata Protocol* is a great fat-burning workout. The idea behind Tabata Protocol is that your body operates at its maximum intensity in short bursts of time with very little rest in between sets. This type of training is ideal for increasing your endurance and burning fat (check out www.en.wikipedia.org/wiki/High-intensity_interval_training for more information).

You can perform nearly any exercise using the Tabata Protocol; in this section, I let you choose a Tabata Protocol workout featuring one of the following: swings, snatches, or renegade rows with two kettlebells. You do 20 seconds of the exercise, followed by a very brief period (10 seconds) of rest. Typically, you perform eight sets total.

Although you may not think doing eight sets of one exercise sounds too hard, the Tabata Protocol workout is extremely challenging; you need to work up to doing eight sets rather than trying to perform eight sets right away. Start with three sets, and gradually work your way up by adding a set or two with each subsequent workout. If you aren't gasping for air after three sets, you need to increase the size kettlebell you're using (see Chapter 3).

You can do your Tabata Protocol workout at the beginning or end of a *light* workout day or as a stand-alone routine. Limit your Tabata Protocol workouts to one or two days a week.

To warm up for this exercise, do three to five stretches from Chapter 5. After you're warmed up, choose one of the workouts in Table 13-4 to get moving.

Table 13-4	Tabata Protocol Workout			
Exercise	*Time for Each Set*	*Number of Sets*	*Rest Period between Sets*	*Reference Chapter*
Two-arm swing	20 seconds	8	10 seconds	6
Snatch on left and right sides (alternating sides)	20 seconds on each side	8 (4 sets on each side)	10 seconds	12
Renegade row with two kettlebells	20 seconds	8	10 seconds	11

When you're finished with your workout, cool down with any three cool-down stretches or Z-Health movements from Chapter 5.

Great Kettlebell Combinations to Try

The combinations in this section (in order from easiest to most advanced) give your workouts even more variety and challenge and also increase the fun factor. Basically, to do each workout in this section, you combine individual kettlebell exercises to make one powerful, difficult, and fluid combination. So why are kettlebell combinations more challenging than single kettlebell exercises? Here are just a few reasons:

✔ You tax all your major muscle groups for a longer period of time than you do with a single exercise.

✔ You hit more muscle groups than you do with a single exercise.

✔ You have to focus longer on what you're doing than you do with a single exercise.

✔ You test your cardiovascular endurance and stamina more than you do with a single exercise.

If you aren't comfortable or proficient in any single exercise mentioned in the following sections, wait until you are before trying the combinations. You don't want to hurt yourself!

The hot potato/Russian twist combo

Both the hot potato and the Russian twist are effective core exercises, so it's no surprise that the challenge for this combo comes from your abdominal endurance and strength (see Chapter 11 for details on the individual exercises).

To do the *hot potato/Russian twist combination,* follow these steps:

1. **Sit on the floor and hold your kettlebell on your left palm, handle facing down; bend your knees and bring your heels off the floor, squeeze your glutes and abs, and keep your knees together.**

2. **Twist your torso to the left and let your eyes follow the movement so that you're looking to the left as you twist (see Figure 13-1a).**

3. **Return to the center, and then, as you twist to the right, pass your kettlebell from your left palm to your right palm, keeping your arms close to the body (see Figure 13-1b).**

When you pass the kettlebell from hand to hand, keep the arc small and in front of your body with your arms close to your rib cage. Make sure your abs are braced and you're breathing properly (as I describe in Chapter 5).

Figure 13-1:
The hot potato/ Russian twist combination.

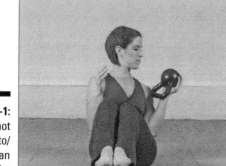
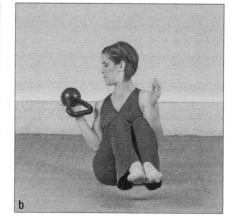

a   b

Perform the combination for one minute; do a total of three sets with a short rest break of 10 to 20 seconds in between sets.

The single-leg dead lift/one-arm row combo

The single-leg dead lift is a superb exercise for increasing your leg and glute strength, challenging your balance, and testing your core strength and stability. Adding the one-arm row to the mix builds even more leg and glute strength, further challenges your balance, and increases the difficulty of the exercise quite a bit. (Turn to Chapter 10 for details on how to do each of these individual exercises.)

To do the *single-leg dead lift/one-arm row combination*, follow these steps:

1. **Stand with your feet slightly apart and your arms down in front of your thighs with your kettlebell in your left hand.**

2. **Lift your right leg off the ground and behind you, take a deep inhale through the nose, and look at a focal point 6 feet ahead of you and down.**

   Maintain a neutral spine as you lift your leg behind you; initiate the movement by pushing your hips back and letting your working (left) knee bend slightly as you do.

3. **Slowly sit back into your hips as you let the left knee bend slightly.**

   Turn to Chapter 4 for details on how to sit back into your hips.

4. **Execute a one-arm row while you're in the single-leg dead lift position, keeping your back in neutral position (see Figure 13-2).**

5. **Return the kettlebell to the bottom position of the row, and then drive through your left heel and use your abs and glutes to stand up tall; put your right foot on the ground.**

Perform five repetitions on each side.

The full Turkish get-up/high windmill combo

I can't imagine putting together two better exercises than the full Turkish get-up (TGU) and the high windmill for a tricky combination that demands core and shoulder stability and strength. You absolutely have to be proficient in each exercise before attempting this combination. Refer to Chapter 7 for proper instruction on the full TGU and Chapter 10 for the high windmill.

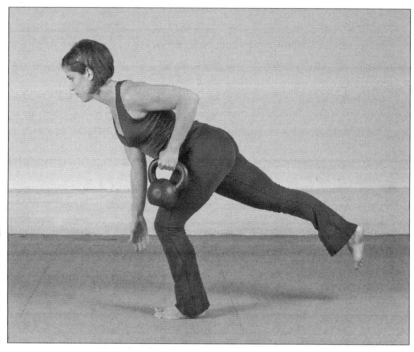

Figure 13-2:
The single-leg dead lift/one-arm row combination.

To do the *full Turkish get-up/high windmill combination,* follow these steps:

1. **Lie face up on the ground and roll onto your left side to get your kettlebell into position with both hands.**

   To get the kettlebell in position, use your left hand to get an underhand grip through the handle of the bell and then place your right hand over your left hand with an overhand grip.

2. **As you roll back onto your back, bring the bell to your chest with both hands, and bend your left knee to a 90-degree angle, keeping your left foot and heel on the floor.**

3. **Press the kettlebell up with your left hand, fully locking out your left elbow; release your right hand.**

4. **Using your right hand to help you, aggressively sit up at a 45-degree angle, keeping your left elbow fully locked out and putting your left foot flat on the floor (with your left knee still bent); then come to a fully seated position.**

5. **Sweep your right leg back and under you, keeping your left elbow fully locked out (see Figure 13-3a).**

   If you perform this step correctly, your body will be in somewhat of a *T* position.

6. **Come to a lunge position with your right knee still on the ground and your left arm pressed overhead in a full lockout position (see Figure 13-3b).**

7. **From the lunge position, stand up tall, pushing through your left heel, and bring your feet together, taking care to keep the left arm up overhead (see Figure 13-3c).**

8. **With the kettlebell overhead in the lockout position and your eyes on the kettlebell, execute a high windmill by positioning your feet according to your ideal windmill stance; push into your left hip as you slowly descend, keeping your left leg straight and bending your right knee slightly if needed, and keep your head in line with your spine as you reach for the middle of your foot with your right hand; then tap the floor with your right hand (see Figure 13-3d).**

   Refer to Chapter 10 for details on how to get into your ideal windmill stance.

9. **Drive through your heels, and, in a controlled motion, stand up tall, still keeping your eyes on the kettlebell and your left elbow locked.**

10. **Finish the Turkish get-up by getting into the lunge position in Step 6 and then working backward through Steps 5 to 1.**

    In Step 5, your leg will sweep forward rather than back.

Perform three total reps on each side, making sure to alternate sides.

Want to take this combo up a notch? Perform all your repetitions on one side before switching sides.

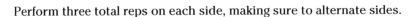

The deck squat/snatch combo

The deck squat itself (see Chapter 10) is a very demanding exercise. Not only do you need the flexibility and strength to get into a rock-bottom squat, but you also need core strength and balance to finish the movement. In addition, the snatch (see Chapter 12) is one of the most taxing and difficult exercises you'll ever do with a kettlebell. Putting these two exercises together makes for one very tough combination.

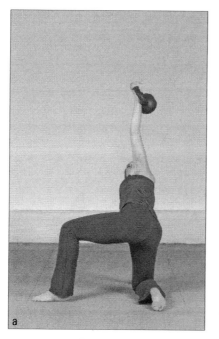
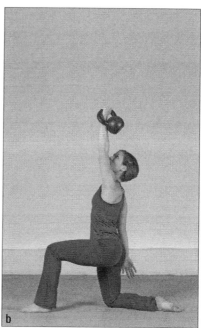
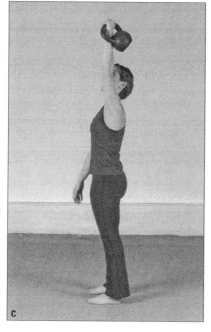
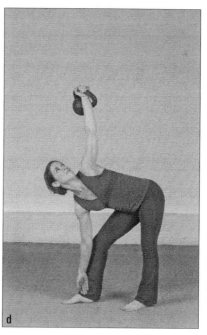

Figure 13-3:
The full
Turkish
get-up/high
windmill
combination.

To do the *deck squat/snatch combo,* follow these steps:

1. **Stand with your feet shoulder width apart, bend your arms, and hold your kettlebell by the horns in front of your body at your chest.**

   Holding the bell by the horns means holding the bell with two hands on either side of the handle.

2. **Reach back with your hips as if you're doing a rock-bottom front squat, and, as you approach the ground, slowly sit back onto your rear end, keeping your arms bent with the kettlebell close to your chest (see Figure 13-4a).**

   Turn to Chapter 8 for details on how to do the rock-bottom front squat properly.

   Take care not to "fall" into this position for risk of hurting your tail bone.

3. **Slowly roll back on your spine, letting your bent legs and feet follow you toward your chest; keep the kettlebell at chest level.**

4. **Use your legs to give you some momentum to fire back up into the rock-bottom squat position, projecting the kettlebell straight out in front of you to act as a counterbalance, and, in one controlled motion, drive back up through your heels to stand up tall.**

5. **Perform a snatch by releasing your right hand from the bell so just your left hand is on the bell (see Figure 13-4b); push your hips back as the kettlebell swings back behind you and drive through your heels to bring the kettlebell up to the top snatch position (see Figure 13-4c).**

6. **Bring your kettlebell back down by corkscrewing the bell down in front of you in one fluid motion, and push your hips back to absorb the bell.**

At the bottom of the snatch (Step 6), grab the bell by the handle again with two hands to repeat Steps 1 through 6 for each repetition. Perform five repetitions on each side.

Man or woman maker

My goal in this book is to try to take some of the intimidation factor out of using kettlebells. After all, kettlebells are a great tool for all fitness levels — as long as you do them correctly. But I simply can't sugarcoat some exercises — and the *man or woman maker* is one such exercise. The exercise's name speaks volumes about its intensity because it certainly challenges your manhood or womanhood!

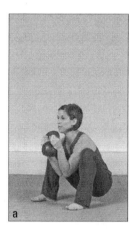
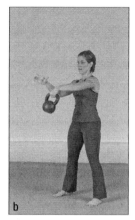

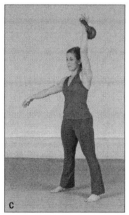

Figure 13-4:
The deck
squat/
snatch
combination.

You need two kettlebells of the same size for this workout, and the kettlebells *must* be at least 26 pounds each; otherwise, they won't be able to support your weight when you do the burpee/renegade row portion of the exercise.

See Chapter 5 for an explanation on how to do a burpee, Chapter 11 for the renegade row with two kettlebells, and Chapter 8 for the squat, the clean, and the press.

To do the man or woman maker, follow these steps:

1. **Stand with your feet shoulder width apart, and position the kettlebells between your feet, handles facing sideways.**

2. **As you push your hips back and reach down to put one hand on each kettlebell, perform a burpee to jump back and down into the plank position and do a push-up (see Figure 13-5a).**

   In other words, from your bent-over position, throw your hips back so you're at the top of a push-up, and then perform a full push-up with your hands on the kettlebells.

3. **After you execute one push-up, perform a renegade row on each side.**

   To perform a renegade row, tighten your abs, glutes, and thighs; with your left hand, lift the kettlebell off the ground and row it toward your rib cage. Your right hand remains steady on the other kettlebell acting as a support for your body. Slowly and in a controlled motion, return the left kettlebell to the ground to the start position; then do the row on your right side.

4. **From the plank position, jump forward and up so that the kettlebells are between your feet and slightly behind you (see Figure 13-5b); your hands stay on the kettlebells as you jump.**

5. **Double clean the kettlebells (see Figure 13-5c).**

   To do so, keep your arms close to your body and rotate your hands inward toward your bells so your thumbs are pointing backward. As you pick up the kettlebells from the ground, drive through your heels to stand upright and snap your hips to clean the kettlebells into the rack position (see Chapter 8 for more details on the rack position).

6. **Keeping the kettlebells racked, perform a rock-bottom squat by sitting back into your hips, letting your knees bend, keeping your spine neutral, and pulling yourself to the ground.**

7. **As you come up from the squat, press the kettlebells up overhead (see Figure 13-5d).**

   See Chapter 8 for details on how to press the kettlebell properly.

8. **Re-rack the kettlebells (refer to Figure 13-5c), bring them back down to the ground between your feet.**

Without taking your hands off the handles, repeat the exercise, beginning with Step 2, for each repetition. Perform five repetitions without resting.

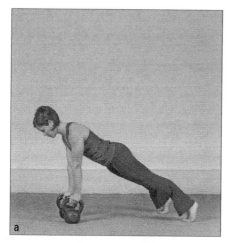
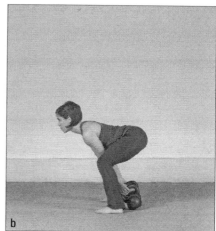
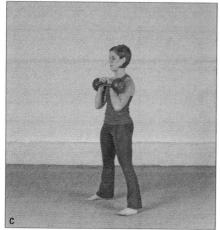
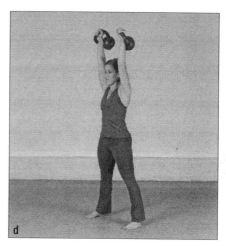

Figure 13-5:
The man
or woman
maker.

Quick but Challenging Combo Workouts

The following combination workouts of 5, 10, and 15 minutes can really boost your energy and help you burn calories during your kettlebell routine. You can add them to your regular workouts for variety or do them as stand-alone workouts; either way, you'll notice results in no time!

To warm up for the five-minute combo workout, do one or two dynamic stretches from Chapter 5, and then perform the exercises in Table 13-5. When you finish all the exercises, cool down with any three cool-down stretches or Z-Health movements from Chapter 5.

Table 13-5	Five-Minute Combo Workout		
Exercise	**Amount of Time in Each Set**	**Number of Sets**	**Rest Period between Sets**
Hot potato/Russian twist combo	1 minute	2	---
Clean/squat/press combo on the left (see Chapter 9)	1 minute	1	30 seconds
Clean/squat/press combo on the right (see Chapter 9)	1 minute	1	30 seconds
Deck squat/snatch combo (alternating sides after each rep)	30 seconds on each side	1	---

To warm up for the ten-minute combo workout, do two dynamic stretches from Chapter 5, and then perform the exercises in Table 13-6. Wrap up with any three cool-down stretches or Z-Health movements from Chapter 5.

Table 13-6	Ten-Minute Combo Workout		
Exercise	**Number of Reps or Time in Each Set**	**Number of Sets**	**Rest Period between Sets**
Full Turkish get-up/ high windmill combo on the left	4 reps	2	10 seconds
Full Turkish get-up/ high windmill combo on the right	4 reps	2	10 seconds
Single-leg dead lift/ one-arm row combo on the left	1 minute	1	---
Single-leg dead lift/ one-arm row combo on the right	1 minute	1	10 seconds

Exercise	Number of Reps or Time in Each Set	Number of Sets	Rest Period between Sets
Deck squat/snatch combo on the left	45 seconds	1	15 seconds
Deck squat/snatch combo on the right	45 seconds	1	15 seconds
Single-leg dead lift/ one-arm row combo on the left	1 minute	1	---
Single-leg dead lift/ one-arm row combo on the right	1 minute	1	---
Deck squat/snatch combo on the left	30 seconds	1	---
Deck squat/snatch combo on the right	30 seconds	1	---

To warm up for the 15-minute combo workout, do three dynamic stretches from Chapter 5, and then perform the moves in Table 13-7. When you finish all the exercises, cool down with any three cool-down stretches or Z-Health movements from Chapter 5.

Table 13-7	15-Minute Combo Workout		
Exercise	**Number of Reps in Each Set**	**Number of Sets**	**Rest Period between Sets**
Full Turkish get-up/high windmill combo on the left and right sides	2 reps on each side	1	30 seconds
Man or woman maker	2	1	30 seconds
Two-arm swing (see Chapter 6)	5	1	30 seconds
Man or woman maker	3	1	30 seconds
Two-arm swing (see Chapter 6)	10	1	30 seconds
Man or woman maker	4	1	1 minute
Two-arm swing (see Chapter 6)	15	1	30 seconds
Man or woman maker	5	1	1 minute

Part IV
Using Kettlebells in Special Situations

The 5th Wave By Rich Tennant

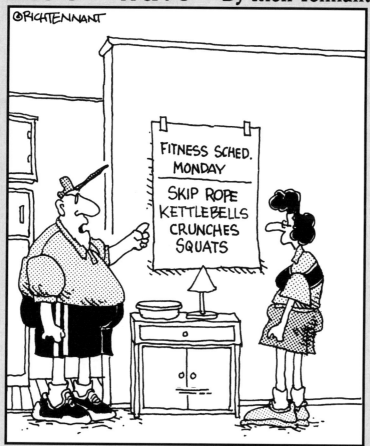

"I AM following the schedule! Today I skipped the rope, then I skipped the kettlebells, then I skipped the crunches."

In this part . . .

Part IV offers kettlebell exercises and routines for those of you who don't fall into the category of the average exerciser. Perhaps you're a young adult, a baby boomer, a senior, or an athlete. Maybe you're in the middle of losing a major amount of weight, or you're just beginning the strength-training phase of your rehab routine. If you fit into any of these categories, you've come to the right place — this part tells you what you need to know to get started with kettlebells. Here, you find lots of recommendations for which exercises are appropriate for your specific situation, as well as a few suggested workout routines to follow. For all you moms-to-be and new moms, turn to Chapter 15 to find out how you can use kettlebells to benefit you and your baby.

Chapter 14

Addressing the Fitness Needs of Young Adults, Boomers, and Seniors

In This Chapter

▶ Knowing the most important differences in your kettlebell routine

▶ Putting together a workout for young adults

▶ Modifying a workout for boomers and seniors

The versatility of kettlebell exercises makes them easy to adapt based on an exerciser's specific needs. Case in point: If you're a young adult (between 13 and 24 years old), a baby boomer (at least 45 years old), or a senior (at least 65 years old), the kettlebell workouts you do will be slightly different from the workouts an average adult between the ages of 25 and 44 does (in other words, if you fit into one of these three groups, don't attempt the workouts in Chapters 9 and 13 just yet). Don't worry, though — strength training has the same benefits for you that it does for the average adult; you just have to go about it a little differently. Just because you're young or, ahem, mature doesn't mean you shouldn't exercise to keep your bones strong, improve your strength level, and challenge your body.

For the first few months of using kettlebells, mastering the basics in Part II of this book will be your main goal. In addition, your workouts will be short but challenging and diverse enough that you won't get bored with them. Plus, you'll see increases in your strength and fitness level almost immediately. This chapter is here to help you get started with your kettlebell routine; it focuses on specific exercises for young adults, boomers, and seniors to use during workouts.

As a young adult, a boomer, or a senior, it's important to get your doctor's approval before you begin a strength-training program. You can even take this book with you to your appointment and dog-ear this chapter to show your doctor exactly what you'll be doing.

Modifying Your Routine to Fit Your Situation

The most important modifications you need to make in your kettlebell routine (compared to that of the average adult exerciser) are

- ✔ **Use light kettlebells:** Women can begin in the 10-pound to 14-pound range, and men can begin in the 14-pound to 18-pound range. (See Chapter 3 for more details on how to pick the right kettlebell.)

- ✔ **Keep kettlebell exercises basic:** Simple is best, so concentrate on mastering the basics and continuing to practice them during your workouts. (Turn to Part II of this book for some great basic exercises.)

- ✔ **Keep workouts short but challenging:** Stick with 15- to 25-minute workouts two to three days per week.

If you fall into the age categories in this chapter but happen to be in peak physical condition, you can jump to the workouts in Chapters 9 and 13 right away, but make sure you follow the guidelines in Chapter 3 for picking the right size kettlebell.

Making Kettlebells Work for Young Adults

Over the years, I've received many calls from parents who love their kettlebell workouts so much that they want to know how they can get their kids involved. Well, this section is for all those parents and their kids.

Basic kettlebell exercises can be a good fit for young adults; much research exists to support the benefits of youth strength training, including building bone strength and muscle tissue, losing weight, building power and endurance for sport-specific activities, and building confidence and motor-fitness performance. As a strength-training exercise routine, kettlebells can be just the workout to help young adults reach their fitness goals.

In the following sections, I provide some important guidelines for young adults who want to start a kettlebell routine. Then I cover the three exercises that should make up that routine: the two-arm swing, the front squat, and the clean and press. I also provide a complete program for young adults to do.

Some special guidelines for young adults

Typically, the parents who ask me whether their kids can use kettlebells want them to strength train as part of their sport-specific training. Whether kids play baseball, softball, or soccer or run track, they're always looking for ways to improve their performance and fitness levels. Adding a kettlebell workout or two to a young adult's weekly exercise routine is a great way to do just that, and the transference of benefits to a specific sport are almost immediate. But even if a young adult doesn't play sports, kettlebells are a good exercise tool for them to consider.

Whether you're a young adult who works out regularly or one who's looking to start an exercise routine for the first time, it's important for you to follow these guidelines when starting to use kettlebells:

- ✔ **Because of the dynamic nature of many of the kettlebell exercises, you need to accurately judge your skill and attention level.** If you can pay attention and follow directions, and if you have good body control and awareness (for example, you can tighten and feel specific muscles), you can proceed with confidence to the basic kettlebell routine in the following section.

  If you have a hard time following directions and/or don't have good body control, kettlebells probably aren't the best workout option for you. You can first master exercises like squats, single-leg dead lifts, pull-ups, sit-ups, and push-ups, which use only your body weight for resistance. Then you can come back to try kettlebells.

- ✔ **If you aren't an accomplished athlete, you need to keep your kettlebell exercises basic so that you get the most out of the workout.** Although you'll most likely find many of the movements in this section natural, you need to focus on doing the basic, foundational moves right so that you can master proper form and avoid injury (and eventually progress to more advanced exercises as you get older).

  If you're a very accomplished athlete, refer to Chapter 16 for specific training guidelines for athletes.

✔ **You need to choose a light, appropriately sized kettlebell with which to start your kettlebell practice.** A 10-to-18-pound kettlebell is an appropriate size for a young adult. The most important part of your training is being able to control the bell's weight with precision (and making sure you aren't flinging it around); using the appropriate size kettlebell will help you maintain this control and precision (refer to Chapter 3 for more information on choosing the right size kettlebell).

✔ **Each of your workouts should last between 15 and 25 minutes, and you should stick with a two-to-three-days-a-week workout schedule.** If possible, alternate the days of your workouts so you get at least a day of rest in between each workout. (If you're an accomplished athlete, refer to Chapter 16 for information on athlete kettlebell training guidelines.)

Note: If you're a parent who's introducing your young adult child to kettlebells, you need to make sure you've mastered the basics and then some before you start teaching your child anything. Ideally, you've been using kettlebells yourself for six months to a year and have at least had your form checked by a Russian Kettlebell Challenge (RKC) – certified instructor or have been training with an RKC during your workouts. If your form and technique aren't up to par, you can't teach anyone else (especially a young adult) how to use kettlebells properly. And, if you really want to help your young adult soar to new fitness heights, have him or her work with a qualified RKC, at least for a session or two. (See Chapter 19 for some tips on working with trainers.)

Great exercises for young adults

The three most beneficial kettlebell exercises for a young adult to do are the two-arm swing, the front squat, and the clean and press. These three exercises, which I explain in the following sections, are basic and should be fairly easy for you to master.

You absolutely must master the techniques and foundational material in Chapters 4 and 5 before you attempt the following exercises; if you don't, you may seriously injure yourself.

The two-arm swing

When you're ready to begin your kettlebell routine, try the two-arm swing first because it's a foundational exercise that teaches your body how to move and use the kettlebell. In addition, the swing is a dynamic exercise that helps you gain strength in your core, butt, and legs and burns calories. To do the two-arm swing, follow the instructions in Chapter 6, and pay careful attention to how your body moves with each swing.

Keep your swings low (chest height or lower), and make sure you fully extend your arms and tighten your thighs, abs, and glutes at the top of the swing (see Figure 14-1a). Forcefully exhale in the top position. In addition, make sure you sit far enough back into your hips at the bottom of the movement (see Figure 14-1b).

Keep the repetition count low in a set (eight or fewer reps); doing so keeps your body from getting too fatigued and helps you avoid losing your form.

Refer to the corrective exercises I describe in Chapter 6, such as the box squat and the face-the-wall squat, if you need help with sitting back into your hips; you can also check out Chapter 4 for hip essentials.

The front squat

The front squat is a great exercise to add to your workout routine when you're young; you'll gain strength in and trim inches from your core, legs, and butt. And, unlike many adults, you'll most likely be able to achieve rock-bottom position without any difficulty; young adults naturally move better than older adults because they aren't inhibited by limited flexibility.

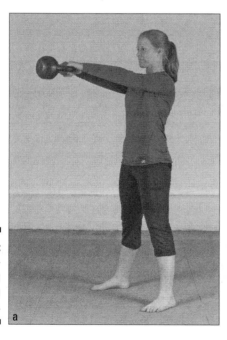 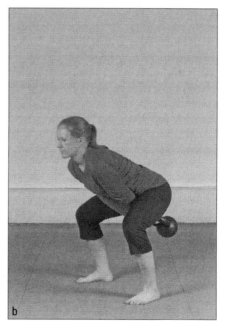

Figure 14-1: The two-arm swing for young adults.

a

b

Chapter 8 explains how to perform the front squat properly. As you move through this exercise, be sure to hold the kettlebell by the horns and keep your spine neutral throughout the exercise (see Figure 14-2a); during the squat section of the exercise, make sure you sit back into your hips as you let your knees bend and descend slowly by pulling yourself to the ground (see Figure 14-2b). Keep the rep count low in each set — five to eight repetitions is enough for this exercise.

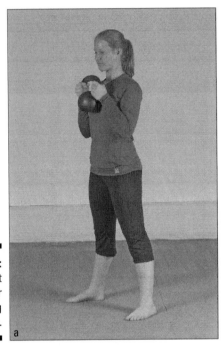 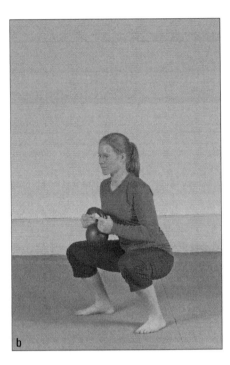

Figure 14-2:
The front squat for young adults.

a   b

Check out the corrective techniques I cover in Chapter 8 (the elevated-heel squat, the band squat, and the box squat) if you have difficulty sitting down into your hips or if you notice problems with your feet or knees during the front squat.

The clean and press

After you master the two-arm swing and the front squat, you can move on to the clean and press, which is a combination of two exercises (the clean and the press) that I describe in Chapter 8. This exercise helps you gain strength in your core and upper body and teaches you how to combine two exercises into one efficient exercise.

Chapter 8 explains how to do the clean and press (take time to master each exercise separately before combining them into one exercise). During the clean and press, make sure you tighten your glutes and abs and stand nice and tall in the top position of the clean (see Figure 14-3a); press your heels through the ground, keep your abs and glutes tight, and lock out your elbow at the top of the press (see Figure 14-3b). In addition, be sure to return your kettlebell to the rack position in a controlled motion.

As with the previous exercises, keep the rep count for the clean and press low. In a set, three to five repetitions on each side is plenty for this exercise.

If you're having trouble mastering the movements in the clean and press, be sure to try out the corrective techniques listed in Chapter 8. Performing the face-the-wall clean, in particular, is a good way to fix clean-specific problems.

Putting together an effective program

Before you do the workout in Table 14-1, make sure to warm up first with two of the warm-up exercises from Chapter 5, like the body weight squat and the halo. After your warm-up, proceed with the workout, doing one set of each exercise, moving through all three exercises before beginning your next set. In addition, make sure you take at least five minutes to cool down, using the cool-down stretches in Chapter 5. This workout should take you approximately 15 minutes; if you add other exercises, your workout should last 20 to 25 minutes.

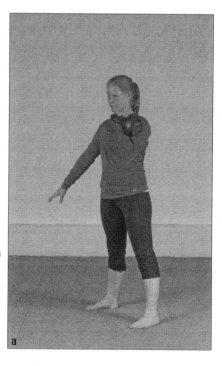
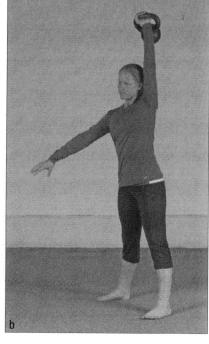

Figure 14-3: The clean and press for young adults.

a

b

Table 14-1	Beginner Youth Workout			
Exercise	Number of Reps in Each Set	Number of Sets	Rest Period between Sets	Reference Chapter
Two-arm swing	5 to 8	3	30 seconds	6
Front squat with kettlebell racked on the left	5	3	30 seconds	8
Front squat with kettlebell racked on the right	5	3	30 seconds	8
Clean and press on the left	3	3	30 seconds	8
Clean and press on the right	3	3	30 seconds	8

If you have other equipment, such as a pull-up bar and a medicine ball, you can mix in other basic exercises, like pull-ups and chin-ups with the bar and sit-up variations with the medicine ball, to create a fun and challenging circuit. In addition, if you aren't doing body weight exercises like pull-ups, you can add the one-arm row from Chapter 10 into your routine. It's an easy exercise to do and will balance nicely with the three kettlebell exercises I describe earlier in the "Great exercises for young adults" section. To add these exercises to your workout, alternate between a kettlebell exercise and a non-kettlebell exercise, like a chin-up, and make sure to take at least a 30-second rest break between each exercise.

Adjusting Kettlebell Workouts for Boomers and Seniors

Active baby boomers and seniors can benefit tremendously from strength training — even more so than the average adult. Typically, by this age, you may have some persistent aches and pains that won't subside (low-back pain or arthritic discomfort, for example), or your balance may not be what it once was. Maybe you've had minor surgeries to repair a knee or shoulder injury and traditional weight lifting isn't appropriate for you anymore. Or, like many of my boomer clients, you've tried every other form of exercise and you're bored, and you want to try something new that makes you feel good. Basic kettlebell exercises may be just the right mix of strength training, cardio, and fun that you're looking for.

In addition to being new and fun, kettlebell exercises benefit your fitness and health levels in less time than traditional weight lifting and exercise, so you don't have to spend hours each week working out in the gym. The fitness and health benefits that kettlebells offer particularly to boomers and seniors include the following (see Chapter 2 for more details on the general benefits of kettlebells):

✔ **Increased muscle mass and increased bone density:** If you don't work out, you lose muscle and bone, which puts you at an increased risk of gaining substantial fat, experiencing musculoskeletal disorders, and having degenerative problems. Sedentary aging leads to five to seven pounds of muscle loss per decade.

✔ **Increased fat loss:** Without a steady workout routine, you stand to gain 20 pounds per decade.

✔ **Increased strength:** This reduces wheelchair use and increases your functional independence.

✔ **Increased functional strength:** This makes your everyday activities less strenuous and more enjoyable.

✔ **Increased balance:** This lowers your risk of falling and seriously injuring yourself.

✔ **Reduced blood pressure:** This reduces the risk of heart diseases and stroke.

✔ **Reduced arthritic symptoms:** Strength training has been proven to reduce the pain of arthritic symptoms, and kettlebells work to strengthen your hands, forearms, and arms with each movement as you grip the kettlebell.

With a list like this one, you owe it to yourself to give a basic kettlebell program a try. In the following sections, I give you some tips on starting a routine modified for boomers and seniors, and I describe the best exercises for the routine.

Some handy advice for boomers and seniors

As a boomer or senior, you need to take note of the following guidelines before you begin your kettlebell routine:

✔ **Start your kettlebell routine by working with a qualified RKC instructor.** If you have any limitations or injuries at all, you really don't have a choice — you need a certified instructor to help make sure you don't overdo it. Even just a few sessions to get you started in the right direction will make a big difference in the results you get from the workout.

If your budget allows, I suggest taking ongoing training sessions or classes because doing so is the best way to make sure you execute the movements correctly. (Flip to Chapter 19 for information on working with a trainer.)

✔ **If you haven't been active for quite some time, begin with a light kettlebell, and work your way up to a more challenging one.** For females, 10 pounds is a good starting weight; for males, 14 pounds works well. If you're currently active and strength training, females can begin with 14 pounds and males with 18 pounds. Choose your kettlebell carefully to make sure it's the appropriate size for you to begin with (refer to Chapter 3 for more tips on choosing the right kettlebell).

✔ **Start with two workouts each week.** If you start by doing just two kettlebell workouts each week, you'll feel and notice a difference within the first few weeks of starting the program. Adding a third workout to your weekly routine will benefit you even more, and the best part is that none of your workouts have to be more than 15 to 25 minutes in length, two to three days per week, with at least a day of rest in between each workout. In other words, you have to spend only 75 minutes working out each week to reap the rewards of kettlebell training.

Excellent exercises for boomers and seniors

As you begin your boomer- or senior-specific kettlebell routine, start with the following three exercises: the two-arm swing, the clean and press, and the low windmill. These exercises give you an excellent foundation on which to build, and after you become proficient with these three basic workouts, you can add other basic exercises from this book into your routine.

Make sure that you've properly mastered the basic forms and techniques in Chapters 4 and 5 before attempting the exercises in the following sections. Otherwise, you're putting yourself at serious risk for injury.

The two-arm swing

The two-arm swing has many benefits, including increased strength and cardiovascular endurance and improved posture. To perform this exercise, follow the steps in Chapter 6.

As you perform the two-arm swing, make sure to keep the height of the swing low (chest height or lower — see Figure 14-4) and to sit back far enough into your hips in the bottom of the movement. Doing so allows you to make sure you aren't using your back to move the kettlebell. Do five to eight repetitions.

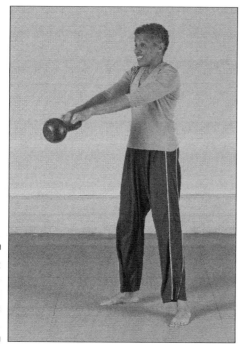

Figure 14-4:
The two-
arm swing
for boomers
and seniors.

The towel swing in Chapter 6 is a good version of the swing to practice to keep your form in check.

The clean and press

The clean and press gives you a lot of bang for your buck. By combining these two moves (the clean and the press), you efficiently and effectively work all the major muscle groups in your body.

Refer to Chapter 8 for instructions on how to perform the clean and press, but be sure to master each exercise separately before combining them into one exercise. When you clean the kettlebell, make sure to keep it close to your body (see Figure 14-5a); when pressing the bell overhead, line your bicep up with your ear and fully lock out your elbow (see Figure 14-5b). Keep your repetition count to three to five on each side to begin with.

Use the face-the-wall clean from Chapter 8 if you end up banging yourself when cleaning the kettlebell; this corrective technique can help you achieve proper form for the clean and press.

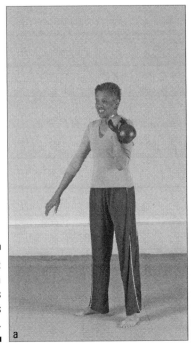
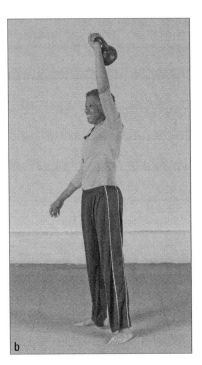

Figure 14-5:
The clean
and press
for boomers
and seniors.

The low windmill

The low windmill is a great exercise to help you gain mobility and flexibility, especially if you have tight shoulders, hamstrings, and hips.

See Chapter 10 for complete instructions on how to properly perform the low windmill. Make sure that you raise your right arm above you, and then push your right hip out and back. Slowly descend to find the kettlebell handle with your left hand; your right arm is still locked above you (see Figure 14-6a). Pick the kettlebell off the floor with your left hand, and with your left arm straightened, glide it along your left leg as you drive through your heels and stand up tall (see Figure 14-6b).

Do three repetitions on the left side without setting down the kettlebell; then set the bell down, switch sides, and repeat for three repetitions on the right side.

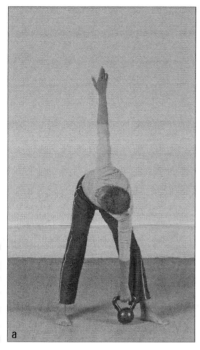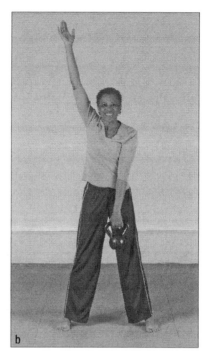

Figure 14-6:
The low windmill for boomers and seniors.

a   b

If you happen to be very flexible, you can try the high windmill in Chapter 10 after mastering the low windmill.

Building a safe program

To do the workout in Table 14-2, first make sure to warm up with two of the warm-up exercises from Chapter 5, like the body weight squat and the downward dog to cobra (pumps) exercise. After your warm-up, proceed with the workout, doing one set of each exercise and moving through all three exercises before beginning your next set. In addition, make sure you take at least five minutes to cool down, using the cool-down stretches in Chapter 5. This workout should take you approximately 15 minutes; if you add in other exercises, your workout should last 20 to 25 minutes.

Table 14-2	Beginner Boomer and Senior Workout			
Exercise	*Number of Reps in Each Set*	*Number of Sets*	*Rest Period between Sets*	*Reference Chapter*
Low windmill on the left	3	1	20 seconds	10
Low windmill on the right	3	1	20 seconds	10
Two-arm swing	5 to 8	3	30 seconds	6
Clean and press on the left	3	3	30 seconds	8
Clean and press on the right	3	3	30 seconds	8

You can add the hot potato from Chapter 11 to your kettlebell program to work your core even more and to challenge your hand-eye coordination. In addition, you can try the one-arm row from Chapter 10 to balance your workout routine; if you need to modify the exercise, use a chair for balance and stability (see Chapter 15 for more on this modified version). Just add these exercises between your swing and clean and press sets.

Chapter 15

Staying Fit during (and after) Your Pregnancy

In This Chapter

▶ Preparing for a prenatal kettlebell workout

▶ Performing moves safely while you're pregnant

▶ Getting back into shape after you deliver

*W*hen I got pregnant with my first child, it seemed natural for me to continue exercising. In fact, I relied on my regular workout routine to help me relieve the tension and aches that accompany pregnancy and weight gain (boy, it hurts when your hips start to widen!). In addition, continuing to strength train kept me feeling strong and fit even though swinging a kettlebell between my legs got increasingly harder as my belly grew. Because of all these benefits and more, I stayed with my routine up until four days before my daughter was born.

Keeping up with my exercise routine during my pregnancy contributed to my smooth labor and quick recovery. I was able to get back into my workouts shortly after my delivery despite my intense sleep deprivation. One reason for my quick jump back into exercise was that my body craved movement and exercise, and, even though I was tired, I was so used to being in a routine that starting one again came easily for me. Best of all, I lost the 45 pounds I gained during my pregnancy within the first three to four postpartum months.

Being pregnant isn't an excuse not to exercise. The benefits of strength training during and after your pregnancy are numerous. You'll relieve aches and pains, gain strength and mobility, have more energy, and sleep better. In addition, you'll recover more easily from labor and delivery and have the energy and strength to keep up with the rigorous demands of motherhood. Even if you haven't started an exercise routine yet, remember it's never too late to start one!

In this chapter, I describe exercises you can do safely during and after your pregnancy, and I provide complete workouts at different intensity levels so you can begin to use kettlebells whether or not you currently strength train.

Gearing Up for a Prenatal Kettlebell Workout

As a mom-to-be, you need to do some preliminary preparation and research before beginning any exercise program, especially a strength-training routine like kettlebells. Although the school of thought used to be that you should never start a new workout program when you're pregnant, doctors and experts are now recommending that women adhere to safe exercise programs during their pregnancies for a variety of reasons.

The program in this section focuses on strength moves that are likely already familiar to your body from your everyday-life activities. I haven't included any extra-dynamic kettlebell exercises because those movements will challenge your body in learning new patterns and movements, which isn't appropriate when you're pregnant. However, if you used kettlebells prior to pregnancy, with your doctor's clearance, feel free to keep the dynamic kettlebell exercises you were doing before your pregnancy in your prenatal routine.

Before you do anything else: Getting your doctor's clearance

It's essential that you consult with your doctor before beginning any prenatal exercise program. If you're having a normal pregnancy, chances are your doctor will recommend that you do some form of exercise, including a strength-training program. The prenatal program I describe in this chapter focuses on strength moves to keep you strong during your pregnancy, and the routines limit dynamic exercises. So let your doctor know that you're going to start a strength-training program, and get the okay from him or her before starting the workouts in this chapter.

Let your doctor know that your kettlebell workouts will be challenging — that you'll be lifting weights as part of this program, that some of the exercises require you to lift the kettlebell over your head, and that your heart rate will be elevated. Discuss with your doctor how many times a week you plan to work out, how long each workout will last, and what size kettlebell you plan to use so your doctor can tell you whether or not the workout is appropriate for your unique pregnancy.

Figuring out which size kettlebell to use

If you're just starting a strength-training routine with this pregnancy program, I recommend beginning with a 5- or 10-pound kettlebell. If you're already using weights in a strength-training program, a 14-pound bell may be a better size for you. If those sizes sound like too much weight for you, consider that your baby is probably going to weigh 7 pounds or more at birth — thus, using anything lighter won't give you much benefit. Plus, you will not only be carrying your newborn around, but most likely a 5-pound diaper bag and maybe another child, as well, so you need to use a weight that challenges you to an appropriate level. (Flip to Chapter 3 for the basics on choosing an appropriately sized kettlebell.)

Replenishing calories after every kettlebell workout

During a 20- to 30-minute kettlebell workout routine, you burn anywhere between 250 and 500 calories. As a result, you need to be diligent about replenishing those calories throughout the day; after all, pregnant women need to stay hydrated and keep a steady supply of nutrients flowing to their growing babies. Protein sources, such as meat, fish, eggs, tofu, high-protein breads, and nuts, are good choices for your postworkout meal. If you're uncertain how to replenish these extra calories, ask your doctor for advice.

I'm pregnant as I write this, and, in addition to my three regular meals a day and several snacks throughout the day, I also add in a small high-protein meal on the days I workout. Sometimes it's as simple as a protein shake, and other times it's a smaller version of lunch or dinner, like a chicken breast, rice, and vegetables.

Core Strength and More: Working Out with Kettlebells during Your Pregnancy

In the following sections, I explain how to do a variety of individual prenatal exercises and show you how to put them together into three comprehensive workouts. All these moves are similar to kettlebell exercises found elsewhere in this book, with appropriate modifications for your ever-changing body. They focus on balance, core strength, and full-body strength. Though these exercises work your cardiovascular system, as well, the intensity is less than a normal (nonpregnancy) kettlebell workout. After all, you don't want to do exercises that leave you short of breath or overheated, neither of which is good for you or your baby.

If you were an active kettlebeller before getting pregnant, keep swings in your routine (see Chapter 6 for more about swings). However, if you're a kettlebell newbie, the swing is best left for your postnatal plan. During pregnancy, your body produces hormones that help prepare your body for labor. As a result of this hormonal change, your joints often become more flexible, and, because the swing is such a dynamic exercise, inexperience could lead to injury. For those of you who have been doing swings as part of your regular routine, I describe how to modify the swing for your pregnancy workout later in this chapter.

Wear comfortable and breathable exercise clothes while working out, and make sure you wear good, supportive shoes. Typically, my students go barefoot or wear flat-soled shoes when working out, but, because you're carrying around additional weight, it's best to wear supportive sneakers for now.

Keeping your balance while strengthening your core

When you're pregnant and your belly is getting bigger and bigger, your center of gravity gets all out of whack and can cause you to become balance challenged. To help you practice and maintain good balance throughout your pregnancy, be sure to include the following balance-specific exercises in your workout routine.

The modified single-leg dead lift

Pregnancy throws your body a lot of curve balls. After you can no longer see your feet, your balance gets thrown off course, and some days you wonder if you'll ever feel your abs tighten again. To help strengthen your core and keep your balance in check, practice the *modified single-leg dead lift* frequently as part of your workout routine. For your prenatal program, include a chair or doorway for balance; check out the original exercise in Chapter 10.

To do the modified single-leg dead lift, follow these steps:

1. **Stand with your feet slightly apart with a chair or doorway positioned on your right side, your left hand holding the kettlebell down at your side, and your right hand on the chair or doorway.**

   Position the chair back or doorway close enough to you that you have only a slight bend in your elbow when touching it.

2. **Lift your right leg a few inches off the ground and behind you; inhale deeply through your nose and look at a focal point on the floor 6 feet in front of you (see Figure 15-1a).**

Keeping your eyes fixed on a focal point not only keeps your neck and spine in proper alignment, but also helps you keep your balance.

3. **Slowly sit back into your hips as you slightly bend your left knee, letting your kettlebell follow your movement (see Figure 15-1b); stop when you feel your belly touch your right thigh.**

   Keep your spine neutral as you push as far back into your hips as you can (see Chapter 4 for details on keeping a neutral spine and sitting back into your hips). Make sure to maintain complete balance and stability throughout the movement.

   Hips first, then knees. Don't forget to lead with the hips — not the knees — while performing this step.

4. **In a controlled movement, drive through your left heel, exhale, and stand up tall, keeping your abs and glutes pinched as you return to the start position in Step 1.**

Perform eight repetitions with the left leg lifted; then switch sides and perform eight repetitions with the right leg lifted.

You should never feel any pain in your back when doing this exercise. If you feel back pain, you aren't sitting back into your hips properly. Your back shouldn't be rounded at any time during this exercise; hinging back into the hips when performing the movement is extremely important, especially when you have a baby in your belly. Refer to the hip and spine essentials in Chapter 4 for complete instructions on sitting back and hinging into your hips.

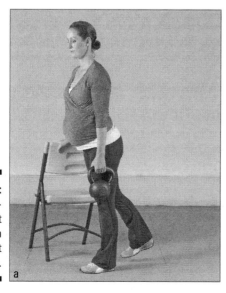 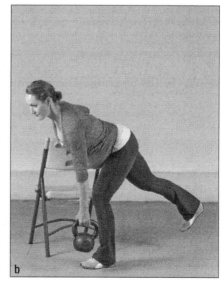

Figure 15-1: The single-leg dead lift modification for pregnant women.

a   b

The modified reverse lunge

Another great exercise for increasing balance and core strength is the *modified reverse lunge*. The lunge has the added benefit of keeping your legs and glutes strong. If you have good balance to begin with, you can do this exercise without using the chair or doorway for assistance, but, if you're uncertain whether you can do this exercise with good form, start with the chair- or doorway-assisted lunge. (You can do a regular reverse lunge by removing the chair or doorway from the following steps.)

To do the modified reverse lunge, follow these steps:

1. **Stand with your feet shoulder width apart, your kettlebell in your left hand, your left arm down at your side, and your chair back or doorway on your right side.**

   Position the chair back or doorway close enough to you that you have only a slight bend in your elbow when touching it.

2. **Step back into a lunge with your right leg, keeping the kettlebell down at your left side, your shoulders back, spine tall, and core tight (see Figure 15-2).**

   Use your right hand on the chair back or doorway to assist you.

3. **Push into your left heel to bring your right leg back to your start position; stand up tall, squeezing your glutes and abs.**

   Don't let your back knee hit the ground when lunging; instead, push into your working heel just before your knee hits the ground to stand back up to your start position.

Perform eight to ten repetitions on the left side (with your right leg lunging); then switch sides and perform eight to ten repetitions on the right side (with your left leg lunging).

Modifying the clean and press for core and upper-body strength

The clean and press (which I introduce in Chapter 8) is a perfect exercise for keeping your core and upper body strong during your pregnancy. However, you may be uncomfortable cleaning a kettlebell into the rack position with a big belly (and big boobs!). To make the exercise a little easier on your joints, try the modification on a stability ball that I describe here; I've used it a lot during my pregnancies.

Perform the press part of this exercise with caution and precision. Because of hormonal changes that affect your joints, you have to be careful not to overextend at the top of the exercise (or else you could end up with an injury). You want to lock out your elbow at the top of the exercise, but make sure not to extend past the lockout position.

If you own a stability ball and can sit and balance on it with ease, the *clean and press on a stability ball* is a great exercise for increasing your core and upper-body strength. Especially if you're experiencing any hip or pelvic achiness and fatigue from your pregnancy, try using a stability ball to make you more comfortable during the clean and press exercise.

The stability ball is a great way to relieve contractions, too, so, if you aren't familiar with this ball, now's the time to get familiar. Just make sure you can sit and balance comfortably on the ball before handling the kettlebell on the ball. If you feel uncertain about sitting on the stability ball and balancing with a weight, back the stability ball up against the wall for more stability.

To do the modified clean and press on a stability ball, follow these steps:

1. **Position yourself on the stability ball so that you're centered with good posture — both feet flat on the ground, shoulders back, and spine tall.**

2. **Place your kettlebell in the rack position on your left side, and release your right hand from the bell so your right arm is out to your side (see Figure 15-3a).**

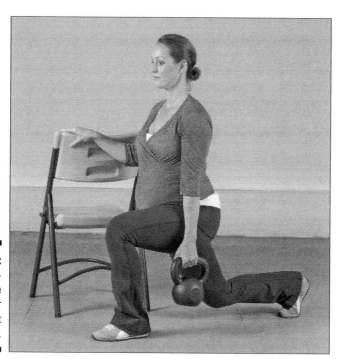

Figure 15-2:
The modified reverse lunge for pregnant women.

To get the kettlebell in the rack position, use an underhand grip to put your left hand through the handle of the bell, and place your right hand over your left to assist you in getting the kettlebell into the left rack position (see Chapter 8 for details).

If you feel unstable or uncomfortable in the rack position, try adjusting your position by making sure your weight is centered on the ball and your spine is tall and extended. Make sure your shoulders aren't rounded or hunched.

3. **Bring the kettlebell down to your left side, keeping your core tight, shoulder in its socket, spine tall, and left elbow close to your side (see Figure 15-3b).**

4. **Use your core to bring the bell back into the rack position described in Step 2.**

    Keep your core tight by using the abdominal bracing and breathing techniques I explain in Chapter 5.

5. **In a slow and controlled motion, press the kettlebell overhead until your left elbow is locked out.**

    Your left bicep should be in line with your left ear, your spine should be tall and your core tight (see Figure 15-3c).

6. **Actively pull the kettlebell back down into the rack position.**

    To pull the kettlebell back into the rack position, actively pull it down by recruiting your lat muscles to help you rather than just bringing it down with your shoulder muscles.

Perform five to eight repetitions on your left side; then switch sides and repeat for five to eight repetitions on your right side.

Making your core and back strong with the one-arm row

The one-arm row is a great exercise for increasing your core and back strength. You can do this exercise by following the steps I describe in Chapter 10. However, if the position doesn't feel good to you because your belly is in the way, do the *modified one-arm* row by using a chair or weight bench to help anchor you.

To use a chair or weight bench to account for your growing belly as you do the modified one-arm row, follow the steps I provide in Chapter 10, but place a chair or bench so that the seat is a few inches from your nonworking hand (the hand opposite the one you're holding the bell with). Place your nonworking hand's palm down on the chair or bench, and use it to anchor you (see Figure 15-4) since you can't comfortably get your elbow on your thigh as you traditionally do in the one-arm row.

Perform eight repetitions on the left side; then switch sides and perform eight repetitions on the right side.

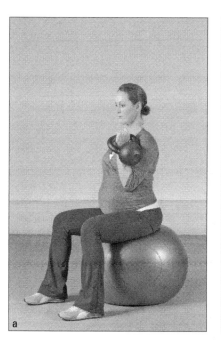

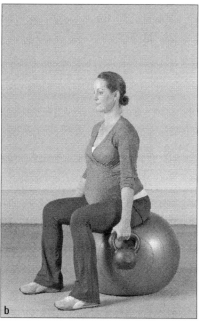

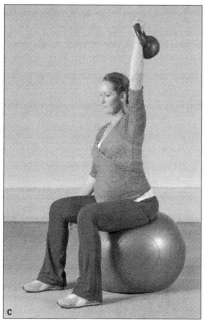

Figure 15-3:
The clean and press on a stability ball.

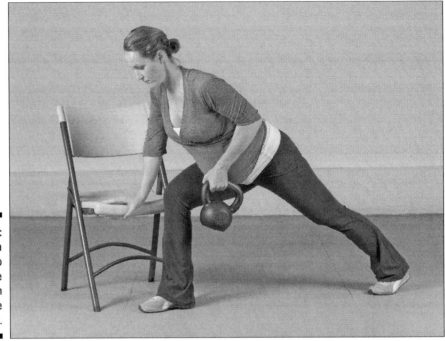

Figure 15-4:
Using a
chair to
make the
one-arm
row more
comfortable.

Keeping your core strong for the big push

After pushing for more than three hours for my daughter's birth (not to mention the four days I spent doing deep abdominal breathing when I was in prelabor), I felt like I had just done three hours of crunches — wow, were my abs sore! Lucky for you (and me!), you can ease the effects of labor and recovery by prepping your core with a variation of the plank position, which is perfect for your growing belly.

If you've done other exercises like yoga or Pilates before, you may be familiar with the plank position already. Basically, the plank exercise requires you to hold your body in a straight line facing the floor while using your elbows and your toes for stability — you have to recruit all your core muscles to hold this position. Even though you don't use a kettlebell for this exercise, it's a highly beneficial exercise to add into your routine to tone and strengthen your abdominal muscles, which are stretched during pregnancy.

If you're still able to perform the plank without assistance, do so. However, as your belly gets bigger, chances are you'll feel low-back strain while performing the traditional plank. Using your knees to support you during the plank is a good way to get the benefit of the exercise without putting added pressure on your back. Just make sure you use a soft floor surface, such as carpet or matting.

To do the *knee-supported plank,* follow these steps:

1. **Kneel on the floor; place both of your arms in front of you, and put your weight into your forearms.**

2. **Position your body in the plank position by shifting your weight forward into your shoulders and forearms so that your core and lower body are even with your upper body (see Figure 15-5).**

   Your butt shouldn't stick up in the air.

3. **Squeeze your glutes, thighs, and abs as you hold this position for 30 seconds to one minute.**

Think about pulling your elbows toward your feet as you hold the plank, and make sure to breathe with natural inhales and exhales during the exercise (see Chapter 5 for more details about breathing right during your kettlebell exercises).

Perform two sets of plank holds, resting as needed between each set by coming into a seated position on the floor.

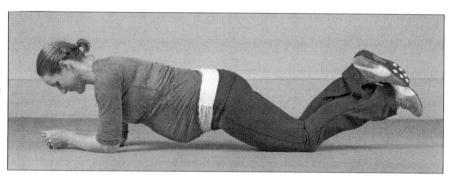

Figure 15-5: The knee-supported plank.

Preparing for labor: Squatting for core, leg, and glute strength

Squats are one of the best exercises you can do to develop core, leg, and glute strength and to prepare your body for labor. Whether you plan to give birth lying down or squatting, you'll need a lot of core and leg strength. Plus, you'll find it much easier to carry around the added weight while you're pregnant if your core, legs, and glutes are strong. Additionally, you'll experience less lower-back pain during and after your pregnancy if you perform squats regularly during your workout routines.

In this section, I describe three squat variations to try, beginning with an easier version and progressing to more advanced versions. Figure out which variation feels right for your body by trying each one.

The chair squat

The *chair squat* is exactly what it sounds like! You simply place a chair behind you and squat toward it. Be sure to use a sturdy chair and place it on a no-slip surface, such as a carpet or mat.

To do the chair squat, follow these steps:

1. **Stand in front of your chair with your feet slightly wider than shoulder width apart, your kettlebell in the left rack position, and your right arm out to your side; take a half or full step forward.**

   To get the kettlebell in the rack position, use an underhand grip to put your left hand through the handle of the bell, and place your right hand over your left to assist you in getting the kettlebell into the left rack position (see Chapter 8 for details).

2. **Push back into your hips, keeping your spine neutral, as you reach back for the chair with your rear end; tap the chair with your rear end (see Figure 15-6).**

3. **Drive through your heels to stand back up tall, pinching your glutes and abs as you do so.**

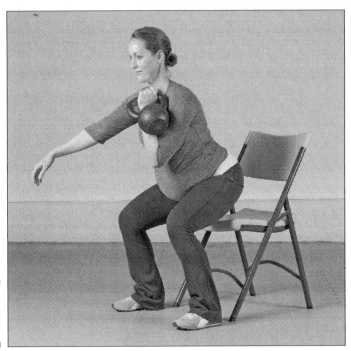

Figure 15-6:
The chair
squat.

Perform five to eight repetitions with the kettlebell racked on the left side; then switch sides and perform five to eight repetitions with the kettlebell racked on the right side.

The box squat

The *box squat* is a very beneficial version of the squat because it helps you sit back into your hips the right way, which, in turn, helps you perform any version of the squat (including the ones you'll do during labor). Just make sure the box you use is meant to hold your weight. You can purchase exercise boxes called *plyometric boxes* in different heights. An 18- to 24-inch box works well for a pregnant woman doing the box squat.

To do the box squat, place your box behind you and take a half or full step forward. Stand with your feet slightly wider than shoulder width apart, your toes pointed slightly out, and your arms down at your sides. Bring your arms out in front of you, and, with your weight on your heels, sit back into your hips, letting your knees bend as you slowly pull yourself to the box. With your weight pushing through your heels and your knees and core stable, drive up to a fully standing position, with your spine tall and glutes pinched (refer to Chapter 4 for complete instructions). Be sure to keep your spine neutral throughout this movement (see Chapter 4 for more information).

Perform five to eight repetitions.

The deep squat

The *deep squat* (or *front squat* as it's also called) is one exercise that many books geared toward pregnant women recommend (check out the sidebar "The deep benefits of squats before labor" to find out why).

To do the deep squat, follow these steps (refer to Chapter 8 for more detailed instructions).

1. **Stand up tall with your feet slightly wider than shoulder width apart, and hold your kettlebell by the horns (with two hands on the handle) close to your body at about chest height.**

2. **Sit back into your hips as you let your knees bend, keeping your spine neutral throughout the movement, and descend slowly by pulling yourself to the ground.**

   Keep the kettlebell in front of you, close to your body, and at chest height throughout the movement.

3. **Without pausing in the bottom position, drive up through your heels, keeping your knees and core stable, to the fully standing position; make sure your spine is tall, and pinch your glutes at the top of the movement.**

Perform five to eight repetitions.

The deep benefits of squats before labor

During my first pregnancy, my doctor gave me a booklet with recommended exercises, and the deep squat was in it. When I went into labor, I realized why the deep squat was such a beneficial exercise to have practiced during my pregnancy. I had a natural birth, so I was free to move about as my body directed me to. After fighting with gravity for more than three hours while trying to "push" my daughter out lying down, I finally realized I needed to squat. I never planned on giving birth in a squat position, but it was what my body directed me to do at the time. Luckily, I was physically prepared to do so (although it was strenuous and challenging) because I had practiced deep squats throughout my pregnancy.

Using additional exercises to keep your core and lower body strong

This section outlines three more kettlebell exercises that will keep you feeling strong and fit during your pregnancy. All three focus on the core and lower body.

The suitcase dead lift modification

The *suitcase dead lift* targets your core, legs, and glutes. Typically, you'd start the suitcase dead lift with your feet together, but, to account for your growing belly, it's fine to keep your feet wider so you can sit back into your hips properly. The movement gets its name because it resembles what you do when you pick up a suitcase (or diaper bag) that's positioned down at your side.

To do the suitcase dead lift, follow these steps:

1. **Stand with your feet a bit closer than shoulder width apart with your kettlebell down at your side in your left hand.**

   Your right hand and arm are at your side.

2. **Keeping your spine neutral, shoulders back, and abs tight, push back into your hips, keeping your weight on your heels as you try to tap the bell down to the floor (see Figure 15-7).**

   Go down only as far as you can to accommodate your belly; try not to twist toward the kettlebell while you perform the suitcase dead lift. Your body will naturally try to do so if your belly is too big and you're trying to touch the floor. It's better to go only as low as you can with good form than to touch the bell to the ground with bad form.

3. **Drive up through the heels to stand up tall, squeezing your abs, glutes, and thighs and keeping the kettlebell down at your side with your elbow locked.**

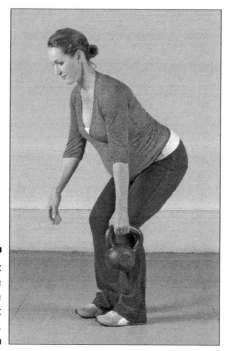

Figure 15-7:
The suitcase dead lift modification.

Perform ten repetitions on the left side; then switch sides and perform ten repetitions on the right side.

The sumo dead lift

I love the *sumo dead lift* as a kettlebell exercise for any routine, but it's especially good to practice when you're pregnant because you don't need to do any modification. Plus, it's an excellent exercise for increasing core, leg, and glute strength.

To do the sumo dead lift, follow these steps:

1. **Stand with your feet slightly wider than shoulder width apart, toes pointed out slightly; hold the kettlebell with two hands in the center of your body (see Figure 15-8a).**

2. **With your spine neutral and abs tight, push back into your hips and keep your weight on your heels; pull yourself down until the kettlebell taps the floor (see Figure 15-8b).**

   Go down only as far as you can to accommodate your belly. Remember it's better to go only as low as you can with good form than to touch the bell to the ground with bad form.

3. **Drive up through your heels to stand up tall, pinching your abs, glutes, and thighs.**

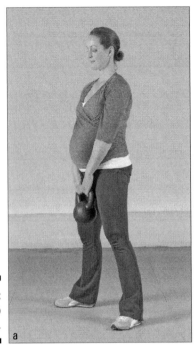
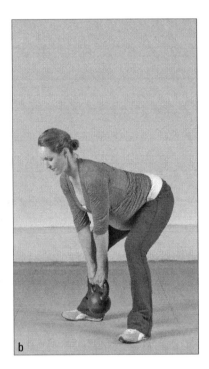

Figure 15-8:
The sumo dead lift.

Perform ten repetitions.

The renegade lunge

Renegade lunges emphasize pushing back into your hips as you move from side to side and then pushing into one leg to complete the movement. Both the traditional, lateral (side-to-side) lunge and the renegade lunge work your core, legs, and glutes, but the renegade lunge is more strength intensive, which is why I focus on it here.

To do the renegade lunge, follow these steps:

1. **Stand with your feet slightly apart, and hold your kettlebell by the horns at chest height (see Figure 15-9a).**

2. **Push back into your hips as you step out to the right side, letting your left knee bend (see Figure 15-9b).**

   When doing the renegade lunge, think about pushing your hips back as if you're trying to duck under a fence or pole.

3. **Push off with a slightly bent right leg (see Figure 15-9c) as it straightens to help you stand up tall and get back into the start position in Step 1.**

   Make sure to pinch your glutes and abs as you stand up tall.

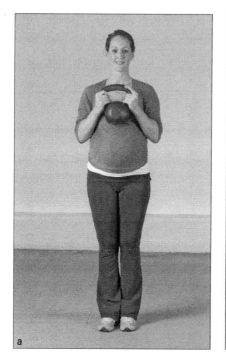
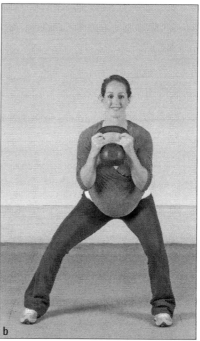

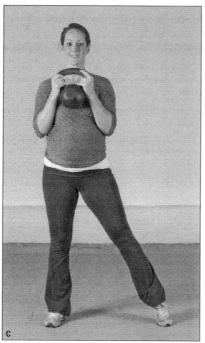

Figure 15-9:
The
renegade
lunge.

4. Repeat Steps 2 and 3 in the other direction (lunging to the left side).

Perform a total of 20 repetitions, making sure to alternate sides in each repetition. Lunging to both sides equals one full repetition.

Trying three complete workouts

Using the exercises illustrated in the preceding sections, I've designed three workouts specifically for pregnant women. I outline these workouts in this section; they advance from easiest to most challenging. These workouts should last 20 to 25 minutes, and you can take breaks as needed. Try to do these workouts consistently two to three days per week to reap their full benefits.

Above all else, listen to your body. One day you may be able to get through a workout with ease, and the next day you may be able to easily complete only a portion of a workout because you're feeling tired. You don't need to push yourself during your pregnancy — your goal is to gain energy and strength from your workouts, not deplete your body. Make sure you have plenty of water close by, and be careful not to get overheated.

Workout 1: Baby steps

Workout 1 eases you into a kettlebell workout routine; be sure to continue this workout until you feel ready to progress to the other two more challenging workouts I describe in this section. Complete two to three sets of the following workout, and rest for no less than 45 to 60 seconds in between each exercise:

- Warm-up: Your choice of dynamic stretches from Chapter 5 and then two knee-supported planks for 30 seconds each
- Exercise 1: Clean and press on a stability ball (five reps on each side)
- Exercise 2: Chair squat, box squat, or deep squat (eight reps)
- Exercise 3: Modified single-leg dead lift (five reps on each side)
- Exercise 4: Modified one-arm row (eight reps on each side)
- Exercise 5: Knee-supported plank for 30 seconds
- Cool-down: Your choice of two to three cool-down stretches from Chapter 5

Workout 2: Getting stronger

If you've progressed through Workout 1 and are ready for more of a challenge, try Workout 2. Complete two to three sets of the following workout, and rest no less than 45 to 60 seconds in between each exercise:

✔ Warm-up: Two Z-Health stretch options from Chapter 5 and then two knee-supported planks for 30 seconds each

✔ Exercise 1: Clean and press on a stability ball (eight reps on each side)

✔ Exercise 2: Suitcase dead lift (ten reps on each side)

✔ Exercise 3: Renegade lunge (20 reps)

✔ Exercise 4: One-arm row (eight reps on each side)

✔ Exercise 5: Renegade lunge (20 reps)

✔ Cool-down: Your choice of two to three cool-down stretches from Chapter 5

Workout 3: Power core

Workout 3 is a good workout to try after you've completed at least one of each of the previous workouts. Complete two to three sets of the following workout, and rest no less than 45 to 60 seconds in between each exercise:

✔ Warm-up: Z-Health stretches from Chapter 5 and then two knee-supported planks for 30 seconds each

✔ Exercise 1: Chair squat, box squat, or deep squat with a press combination (ten reps on each side; see Chapter 8 for instructions on how to do the press)

✔ Exercise 2: Supported-knee plank for 30 seconds

✔ Exercise 3: Sumo dead lift (ten reps)

✔ Exercise 4: Chair squat, box squat, or deep squat with a press combination (ten reps on each side)

✔ Exercise 5: One-arm row (eight reps)

✔ Cool-down: Your choice of two to three cool-down stretches from Chapter 5

Powering Up with Postnatal Kettlebells

After you have your baby and your time is no longer your own, it becomes difficult to find time in your day to exercise. Moms are incredibly busy, and exercise usually gets pushed to the back burner. You may also feel guilty spending any extra time you do have on yourself instead of with your family. But guess what? Kettlebells are a great workout for busy moms because, for one, you can do your routine at home with one small piece of equipment (the kettlebell, of course!). Secondly, the workouts are short, intense, and effective. These days, in the time it takes for my husband to feed my daughter breakfast, I can get in a solid kettlebell workout at home. If you don't have that kind of time available, try the workout routines that use baby as your resistance.

Mix up the workouts in the following sections as your hectic life allows you to, and, of course, be sure to have your doctor's clearance before you start any regular postnatal exercise routine.

The key to being successful with your exercise routine is to be flexible about where and when you work out. Before having a baby, I had to work out first thing in the morning; otherwise, it didn't happen. Now, if I can't get in my early morning workout, I remain flexible enough to just let it happen when it does. If you have one (or two) of those off weeks, don't worry. Just pick up your routine as soon as you can, and don't beat yourself up about it. Being a mom is hard work!

Always keep your baby at a safe distance (and not facing you) when you use a kettlebell.

Before you begin: Getting your doctor's clearance for a postnatal workout

Make sure to get the green light from your doctor before starting the routines outlined in the following sections. Typically, doctors want you to wait six weeks before strength training after delivering your baby. If you had a C-section, it's a good idea to stay away from any ab-specific exercises until your incision has healed — sometimes this healing process can take up to three months. The great thing about kettlebells is you can get plenty of core work from a few basic exercises that will tone that mommy tummy in no time — without having to do sit-ups or ab-specific exercises (see the next section).

After you feel ready to progress and have talked to your doctor about starting a workout routine, use the workouts I describe throughout this chapter (and book) to get the ultimate post-baby body. If you aren't sure whether you're ready to move into a regular workout routine, ask your doctor for advice.

Great exercises for strengthening your pelvic floor muscles

I'm sure you've read about doing Kegel exercises to strengthen your pelvic floor muscles after having a baby. They're an effective way to tighten up the muscles that stretched out during childbirth. But who has time to do them? I mean, I don't know about you, but when my baby goes to sleep at night, the last thing I remember to do is my Kegel routine! Don't lose hope, though — three particular kettlebell exercises help you strengthen your pelvic floor muscles without doing Kegels: the two-arm swing (see Chapter 6), the front squat (see Chapter 8), and the clean and press (see Chapter 8).

Necessity is the mother of (kettlebell routine) invention

When my daughter was first born, I was naïve enough to think my workout routine wouldn't change. So when I started back into my kettlebell routine, I toted her along in her car seat to my gym, Iron Core. It just so happened there were five of us new moms at the gym who wanted to get back into shape, so I created a Mighty Mom's class. We got together a few days a week with our babies (who watched from a safe distance) to do our kettlebell workouts. Then, sure enough, a couple of our babies became mobile — and that was the end of bringing them to the gym and expecting them to sit and watch us for 30 minutes!

But we still needed to work out, so I created a stroller-based kettlebell workout that burns mega calories in only 30 minutes — just enough time for Mom to get in her workout and for baby to be pushed around the park without fussing. (The appendix has my contact information if you want to know more about this workout.) On the days when I just couldn't get out of the house, I used several key kettlebell exercises and created a workout using baby as resistance. My daughter loves doing these exercises with me, and, at least, I get in some type of exercise on the days when I can't fit in my regular kettlebell workout.

During any of the workouts in the following sections, take the time with each repetition to focus on squeezing and tightening your pelvic floor muscles, which you should be doing whether you're pregnant or not because it's part of proper kettlebell form. If you aren't sure what it feels like or how to do so, visualize pinching a coin between your cheeks and simultaneously tightening your pelvic floor muscles to stop yourself from urinating. Squeeze and tighten your pelvic floor muscles at the top of each rep, and, by the end of your workout, you'll have done all the Kegels you need to do for the day.

Three at-home kettlebell workouts

The following at-home workouts are designed for women who have recently given birth and, with their doctor's clearance, are ready to start working out. The workouts are short but intense and are perfect for the tired and busy mom. The goal is to complete three sets, but if you can get through only one or two, that's okay, too. As time goes on and you continue to recover from your pregnancy and delivery, you'll be able to complete the workouts.

Use the prenatal guidelines I provide earlier in this chapter for choosing your kettlebell size (see the section "Figuring out which size kettlebell to use"). Try to do the workouts two to three days per week; start with Workout 1 and then move on to Workouts 2 and 3 when you feel ready for more of a challenge. Cool down with any three cool-down stretches or Z-Health movements from Chapter 5.

Workout 1: Baby steps

Workout 1 is designed to get your body moving again and ease you back into a workout routine. Complete three sets of the following workout in 20 to 25 minutes, and rest no longer than 30 seconds in between exercises:

- ✔ Warm-up: Three Turkish get-ups on each side (see Chapter 7)
- ✔ Exercise 1: Two-arm swing (ten reps; see Chapter 6)
- ✔ Exercise 2: Front squat with kettlebell by the horns (eight reps; see Chapter 8)
- ✔ Exercise 3: One-arm row (ten reps on each side; see Chapter 10)
- ✔ Exercise 4: Two-arm swing (ten reps; see Chapter 6)
- ✔ Exercise 5: Clean and press (five reps on each side; see Chapter 8)

Workout 2: Getting stronger

If you're getting rest and feeling stronger, continue progressing with Workout 2. Complete three sets of the following workout in 20 to 25 minutes, and rest no longer than 30 seconds in between exercises:

- ✔ Warm-up: Four low windmills on each side (see Chapter 10)
- ✔ Exercise 1: Alternating swing (ten reps; see Chapter 6)
- ✔ Exercise 2: Tactical lunge (20 reps; see Chapter 10)
- ✔ Exercise 3: Squat and press combo (eight reps on each side; see Chapter 8 for instructions on how to do these two exercises)
- ✔ Exercise 4: One-arm row (ten reps on each side; see Chapter 10)
- ✔ Exercise 5: Russian twist (20 reps; see Chapter 11)

Workout 3: Power core

When you're ready to progress to Workout 3, you're close to being able to resume your regular workout routine. After this workout becomes easy to get through, consider challenging yourself by referring to the workouts in Chapters 9 and 13. Complete three sets of the following workout in 25 to 30 minutes, and rest no longer than 45 seconds in between exercises:

- ✔ Warm-up: Four Turkish get-ups on each side (see Chapter 7) and two sets of ten two-arm swings (see Chapter 6)
- ✔ Exercise 1: Clean/squat/press combination (ten reps on each side; see Chapter 13)

 ✔ Exercise 2: One-arm swing (ten reps on each side; see Chapter 6)

 ✔ Exercise 3: One-arm row (eight reps on each side; see Chapter 10)

 ✔ Exercise 4: Sumo dead lift (15 reps; see the section "The sumo dead lift")

 ✔ Exercise 5: Two-arm swing (15 reps; see Chapter 6)

 ✔ Exercise 6: Hot potato/Russian twist combo (20 reps; see Chapter 13)

Baby as your bell: Using your baby as resistance

On the days when baby just won't let you get in a kettlebell workout or when you're too tired to do so, the baby-as-your-bell workout is a good alternative. In addition, the baby-as-your-bell exercises are great for working up to the kettlebell workouts in the previous sections. This workout is based on basic kettlebell exercises that work your core, legs, and glutes. The best part of this workout is that your baby is in your arms where he or she loves to be!

In the following sections, I describe the exercises you can do with your baby as resistance, and I provide three workouts at different fitness levels for you to try.

You can use a Moby Wrap or Baby Bjorn to keep your baby secure while doing the majority of these exercises.

The chair squat

To do the chair squat with your baby as resistance, follow the steps from the earlier section "The chair squat," but keep your baby secure at your chest by wrapping one arm around her chest and the other arm under her groin — hold tight (see Figure 15-10). Repeat for 10 to 15 reps.

The renegade lunge

To do the renegade lunge with your baby as resistance, follow the steps from the earlier section "The renegade lunge," but have baby secure at your chest (see Figure 15-11). Perform 20 reps.

The Russian twist

To do the Russian twist with your baby as resistance, follow the steps for the Russian twist in Chapter 11, but have your baby in your arms (see Figure 15-12). Perform 20 total reps.

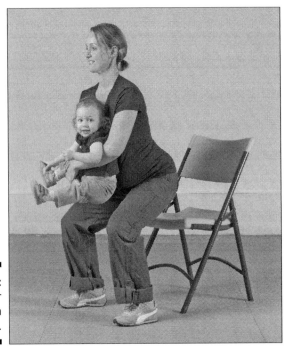

Figure 15-10:
The chair squat with baby.

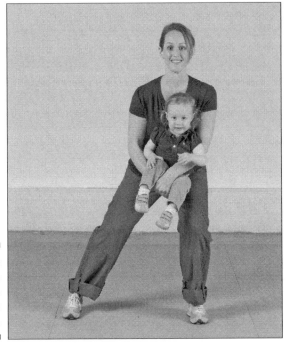

Figure 15-11:
The renegade lunge with baby.

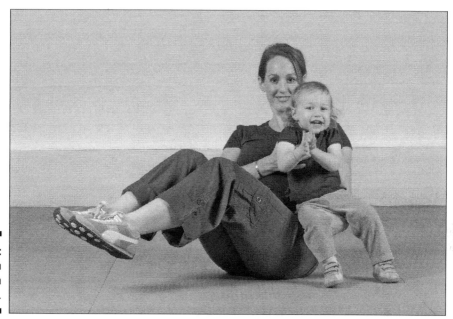

Figure 15-12:
The Russian twist with baby.

The baby swing

To do the baby swing, follow these steps:

1. **Stand with your feet a little more than hip width apart; hold baby securely with two hands at your chest with her weight distributed evenly on both sides.**

2. **Inhale and tighten your abs; push back into your hips as you slowly lower baby toward the ground (see Figure 15-13).**

3. **Drive up through your heels, push your hips forward, tighten your glutes, and bring baby back to the start position.**

Repeat for 15 reps.

The farmer lunge

To do the farmer lunge with your baby as resistance, follow these steps:

1. **Stand with your feet a little more than hip width apart; hold baby securely with two hands at your chest with her weight distributed evenly on both sides.**

2. **Step to the left with your left leg, letting it bend while keeping the right leg straight (see Figure 15-14); keep baby close to your chest.**

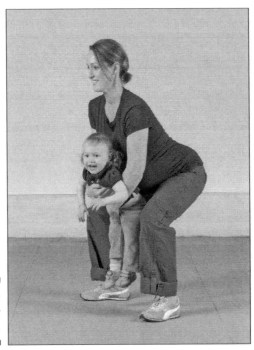

Figure 15-13:
The baby
swing.

3. **Sit back into your hips, and return to center by pushing off with your left leg (into your left heel).**

4. **Repeat Steps 2 and 3 on the right side.**

Perform a total of 20 repetitions, making sure to alternate sides with each repetition.

The single-leg dead lift

To do the single-leg dead lift with your baby as resistance, follow the steps for the single-leg dead lift that I provide in Chapter 10, but have baby secure at your chest (see Figure 15-15). Perform eight reps on each side.

The deep squat

To do the deep squat with your baby as resistance, follow the steps I provide in the earlier section "The deep squat," but have baby secure at your chest (see Figure 15-16). Perform ten repetitions.

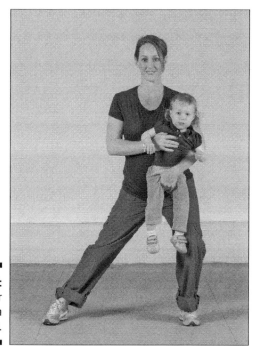

Figure 15-14:
The farmer lunge with baby.

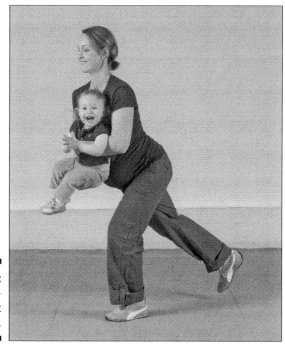

Figure 15-15:
The single-leg dead lift with baby.

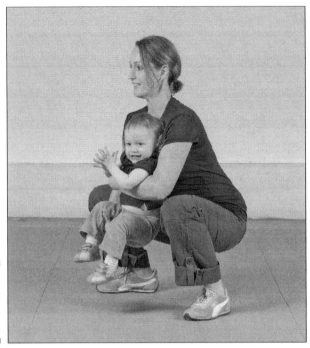

Figure 15-16: The deep squat with baby.

The lunge with rotation

To do the lunge with rotation using your baby as resistance, follow these steps:

1. **Stand with your feet together and baby secure at your chest with your weight evenly distributed.**

2. **Step back into a lunge with your right leg and slowly twist to your left; keep baby close to your chest (see Figure 15-17).**

3. **Push into your left heel to bring your right leg back to the start position in Step 1.**

4. **Repeat Steps 2 and 3 by stepping back with the left leg.**

Perform a total of 20 repetitions, making sure to alternate sides with each repetition.

The baby get-up

To do the baby get-up, follow these steps:

1. **Lie on the ground with your baby secured at your chest; have one hand on each side of her torso.**

2. **Bend your left knee at a 90-degree angle, keeping your left foot on the ground and your right leg straight.**

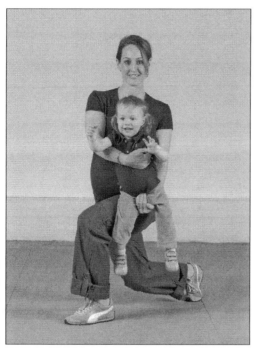

Figure 15-17:
The lunge
with rotation
with baby.

3. **Sit up without bringing your left heel off the ground, making sure to pinch your glutes and engage your abs (see Figure 15-18).**

4. **Keep your abs and your glutes tight as you slowly lower yourself back down.**

Repeat for five reps on the left side; then switch your leg positioning and repeat for five reps on the right side.

Putting the moves together in three complete workouts

For each of the following baby-as-your-bell workouts, try to finish in 20 minutes with little or no rest until you've completed three rounds. Begin with Workout 1 and progress to Workouts 2 and 3 when you feel ready to do so. Cool down with any three cool-down stretches or Z-Health movements from Chapter 5.

For Workout 1, Baby steps, do three sets of the following routine:

- ✔ Warm-up: Two baby get-ups on each side
- ✔ Exercise 1: Chair squat (10 to 12 reps)
- ✔ Exercise 2: Renegade lunge (ten reps total, alternating sides)
- ✔ Exercise 3: Russian twist (ten reps)

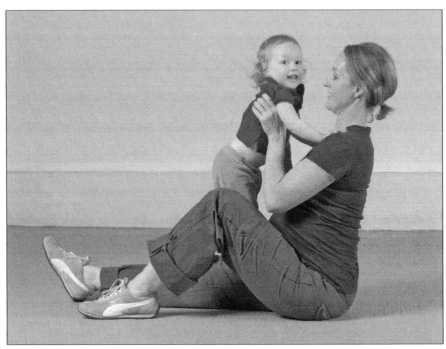

Figure 15-18:
The baby
get-up.

For Workout 2, Getting stronger, do three sets of the following routine:

- ✔ Warm-up: Four baby get-ups on each side
- ✔ Exercise 1: Baby swing (ten reps)
- ✔ Exercise 2: Farmer lunge (20 reps, 10 on each side)
- ✔ Exercise 3: Single-leg dead lift (eight reps on each side)
- ✔ Exercise 4: Russian twist (15 reps)

For Workout 3, Power core, do three sets of the following routine:

- ✔ Warm-up: Russian twist (20 reps)
- ✔ Exercise 1: Deep squat (20 reps)
- ✔ Exercise 2: Lunge with rotation (ten reps on each side)
- ✔ Exercise 3: Farmer lunge (20 total reps, 10 on each side)
- ✔ Exercise 4: Five baby get-ups on each side

Chapter 16

Kettlebell Training for Athletes of All Levels

In This Chapter

▶ Doing exercises appropriate for high-level and recreational athletes

▶ Setting up a workout program for weekend warriors

Kettlebells are a perfect training tool for athletes of all levels. Whether you're a high school, college, or professional athlete or a recreational athlete (who competes in local amateur sports leagues), you can use the kettlebell to improve your overall athleticism as well as the specific skills you use in your sport. The benefits of kettlebell training for high-level and amateur athletes include the following:

✔ Efficient and effective kettlebell workouts are easy to add to your current weight-training routine.

✔ The powerful, dynamic exercises mimic movements in your sport (which means they'll help you perform better).

✔ Kettlebell exercises lead to increases in both cardiovascular and muscular endurance.

✔ Kettlebells strengthen joints and muscles, which makes injuries less likely to occur.

No matter what kind of athlete you are, incorporating just three simple kettlebell exercises into your training routine will make a big difference between you and your competition, as you find out in this chapter. In addition, weekend warriors (folks who like to work out casually a couple of times each week) will surely find the appeal in the quick and intense kettlebell workouts that get results with only two workouts a week. If you just can't fit in workouts during the week, consider trying the weekend-warrior program in this chapter, which outlines the kettlebell exercises that give you the most bang for your buck.

Kettlebells for High School, College, Professional, and Recreational Athletes

If you're an athlete with a demanding playing or competing schedule, you probably don't have much time for anything but playing and practicing during the season. Your strength and conditioning coach has most likely given you a very structured exercise routine that includes exercises like squats, presses and rows, and plyometric, agility, and full-body weight training. But if you want to include more dynamic and explosive versions of these exercises in your training routine, the kettlebell exercises in this section can help get you started; just be sure to follow the kettlebell training guidelines I provide, too.

And don't forget that recreational athletes can also benefit from kettlebell training! As you find out in this section, you can use the same exercises as high school, college, and professional athletes; your kettlebell training schedule is just a little different.

Setting up a training schedule

One reason why kettlebell training is so appealing to athletes of all levels is that it's highly effective and efficient. If you're a high school, college, or professional athlete, you need to spend most of your time practicing your sport, not working out, so you'll find the high effectiveness of kettlebells especially advantageous. After all, you need to be strong and fit, as well as highly skilled, to excel at your sport — and that's where kettlebells can help. You can easily work kettlebell exercises into your current training routine, or you can use them as a stand-alone weight-lifting program with plyometric, agility, and body weight training. After you begin putting kettlebell exercises into your training routine, you'll feel more powerful and have more endurance, and your overall performance in your sport should noticeably improve. (As an example, your vertical leap can improve considerably just from including swings in your training routine.)

Because the intensity of kettlebell training exceeds that of most traditional weight-lifting programs, making sure you don't overtrain is important. Use the following guidelines to make sure you don't overdo it:

- ✔ **Off-season:** Do four to six kettlebell workouts per week.

- ✔ **Preseason:** Do three to four kettlebell workouts per week.

- ✔ **In-season:** Do one or two kettlebell workouts a week, and don't exceed 30 minutes per workout.

- ✔ **Postseason:** Do one to three kettlebell workouts a week.

All the same benefits that apply to high school, college, and professional athletes apply to recreational athletes, too. The only difference for recreational athletes is that they probably don't have as demanding of a training schedule and can fit in more kettlebell workouts during the week. In that case, use the exercises in the next section to begin your kettlebell training, and follow a regular kettlebell training program of two to four days each week to maximize your results.

Trying three great kettlebell exercises

Including kettlebells in your training routine doesn't have to take up a lot of extra time, although learning how to do the exercises properly does take some commitment. After you master the exercises in this section, along with the basics in Part II, you can easily add new exercises to your workout to keep your body challenged — power exercises like the snatch (see Chapter 12) are especially effective for athletes.

An effective kettlebell training program keeps you strong and healthy and can help you prevent injury while you're playing your sport. But you must get instruction from a qualified Russian Kettlebell Challenge (RKC)–certified instructor to ensure you don't get hurt when beginning the exercises. In the appendix, I provide you with a Web link to a list of RKCs by state, some of whom specialize in working with athletes and will even travel to train your team alongside your strength and conditioning coach. Working with an RKC is the best way to begin your training routine so you get the maximum benefit from the training tool and stay healthy.

I recommend starting your training with the two-arm swing, the clean/squat/press combination, and the renegade row with two kettlebells. Before you perform the exercises in the following sections, stay safe by checking out the spine and hip essentials in Chapter 4 and the methods for breathing properly in Chapter 5.

Before executing any of the exercises, make sure you warm up properly. To quickly prepare your body for the following kettlebell exercises, do two or three of the stretches I describe in Chapter 5. In addition, use the cool-down suggestions I offer in Chapter 5 after you finish your workout.

The two-arm swing

The *two-arm swing* is one of the most powerful and dynamic of all the kettlebell exercises. Because it's the cornerstone of kettlebell training, you want to practice this exercise first and practice it well. The swing builds both muscular and cardiovascular endurance and targets the hamstrings, glutes, and core muscles. It also shows your body how to generate maximum power from your hips and glutes. Don't be surprised if you can jump higher, run faster, hit farther, and feel more powerful after introducing swings into your routine.

See Chapter 6 for the details on how to properly execute the two-arm swing. Here's a quick rundown: Swing the kettlebell behind you (like you're hiking a football; see Figure 16-1a), and aggressively snap your hips forward as you stand up tall; drive through your heels, extend your spine, and squeeze your thighs, glutes, and abs as you bring your arms and kettlebell to chest height (see Figure 16-1b).

Perform ten repetitions of the two-arm swing.

The clean/squat/press combination

Undoubtedly you've done the clean, the squat, and the press with a barbell or dumbbell as part of your workout routine, but doing these exercises with the kettlebell gives your body a whole new challenge. The center of gravity and versatility of the kettlebell are markedly different than those of a barbell or dumbbell. You move more dynamically with the kettlebell, and, as a result, your core muscles and major muscle groups are continually challenged to control the weight throughout the movements. This extra challenge helps your body get even stronger and more prepared for your sport.

If you don't have time to do a full, well-rounded kettlebell program, combine the *clean, squat,* and *press* as I do here. Each of these exercises taxes your major muscle groups and keeps your heart rate up. In addition, the movements in these exercises are typically exactly what an athlete needs to develop power while maintaining agility.

Refer to Chapter 8 for details on how to perform each of these exercises individually; Chapter 9 has the scoop on combining them into one smoothly flowing exercise. Here are the three basic moves:

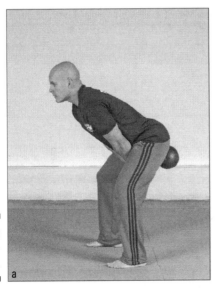 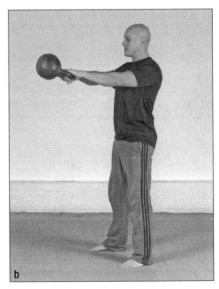

Figure 16-1:
The two-arm swing.

a

b

1. **Clean the kettlebell into the rack position on your left side by driving through your heels and snapping your hips, ending up with a tall spine and your right arm at your side (see Figure 16-2a).**

2. **With the kettlebell in the rack position, descend into the rock-bottom squat position by sitting back into your hips and bringing your rear end as close to the ground as you comfortably can while maintaining a neutral spine (see Figure 16-2b).**

3. **As you drive your heels through the ground to come up from the bottom of your squat, use your whole body to press the kettlebell up into a fully locked out military press (see Figure 16-2c).**

Perform five repetitions of this combo on the left side, and then either set the kettlebell down or take an extra swing to switch sides (refer to the alternating swing in Chapter 6 for instructions on how to do so); perform five repetitions on the right side.

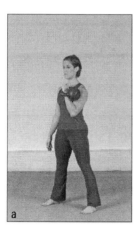
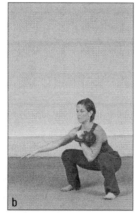
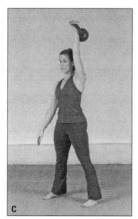

Figure 16-2:
The clean/
squat/press
combination.

The renegade row with two kettlebells

Even though you need to buy two kettlebells of the same size for the *renegade row with two kettlebells,* the benefits you get from it are well worth the investment. This exercise is one of the best in terms of building core and back strength and body control and stability. No matter what sport or athletic activity you're involved in, having a resilient and strong core is one of the keys to performing optimally and staying off the injured list.

Refer to Chapter 11 for all the details on how to perform the renegade row with two kettlebells. Here are the basics:

1. **Begin in a plank or push-up position with your kettlebells shoulder width apart, your hands positioned on the kettlebell handles, your shoulders positioned directly over your hands, your hips square, and your arms straightened (see Figure 16-3a).**

2. **Tighten your abs, glutes, and thighs; with your left hand, lift the kettlebell off the ground and row it toward your left hip as you push your right hand straight down onto the handle of your right kettlebell to stabilize you (see Figure 16-3b).**

Perform ten total repetitions (five on each side), alternating sides after each row.

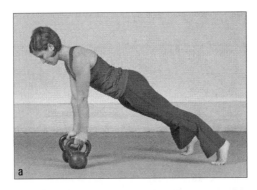

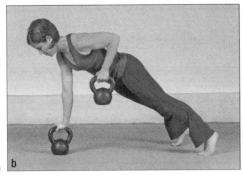

Figure 16-3: The renegade row with two kettlebells.

Kettlebells for Weekend Warriors

If your schedule allows you to weight train only on weekends, you can adopt a Saturday/Sunday kettlebell training routine. If you decide to go the route of the weekend warrior, you need to make sure you don't overdo it by using the right combination of exercises (otherwise, you'll feel exhausted during the rest of your week). I note some great exercises and combinations to do and outline some sample routines in the following sections to help you get started.

Essential exercises and combinations

To get the most bang for your buck, start your weekend-warrior routine by trying the exercises in the previous section: the two-arm swing (see Chapter 6), the clean/squat/press combination (see Chapters 8 and 9), and the renegade row with two kettlebells (see Chapter 11).

After you master these three exercises, you can add the single-leg dead lift/one-arm row combination and the man maker or woman maker. By focusing your training time on these effective combinations, which I describe in the following sections, you accomplish in your two weekend training sessions what most people typically do in four training sessions.

The single-leg dead lift/one-arm row combination

The single-leg dead lift/one-arm row combination is an exercise that challenges your balance and core stability and works your hamstrings, glutes, abs, and back. You need to master the correct form for each of these two exercises before you attempt the combination. Refer to Chapter 10 for how to perform these individual exercises properly. After you know how to do each exercise individually, use the combination to get the job done in half the time! Chapter 13 explains in detail how to put together the two movements in one smooth combination. Here are the basics:

1. **Standing with your feet slightly apart and your arms down in front of your thighs with your kettlebell in your left hand, lift your right leg off the ground and behind you, take a deep inhale through your nose, and look at a focal point 6 feet ahead of you and down.**

   Maintain a neutral spine as you lift your leg behind you; initiate the movement by pushing your hips back and letting your left knee bend slightly as you do.

2. **Execute a one-arm row while you're in the single-leg dead lift position, keeping your back in neutral position (see Figure 16-4).**

3. **Return the kettlebell to the bottom position of the row, and then drive through your left heel, using your abs and glutes to stand up tall; put your right foot on the ground.**

Perform five repetitions on the left side, and then set down the kettlebell to switch sides; perform five repetitions on the right.

The man or woman maker

If you're a true weekend warrior, you need to include this combination of four kettlebell exercises and one body weight exercise in your routine. The combination consists of

✔ The burpee (see Chapter 5)

✔ The renegade row with two kettlebells (see Chapter 11)

✔ The squat, the clean, and the press (see Chapter 8 for all three exercises)

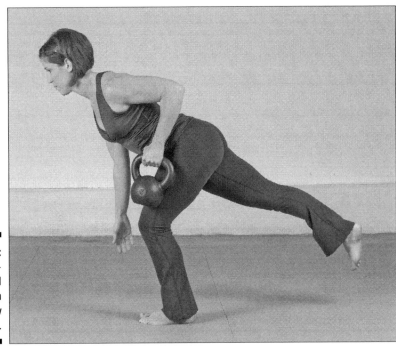

Figure 16-4:
The single-leg dead lift/one-arm row combination.

The good news is that you don't have to do many repetitions to see (and feel) the effects of this intense exercise. The bad news is that each repetition takes a little more time than you may be used to — five times the amount of time a single exercise takes, which means each rep will likely take you at least one minute to complete.

To do the man maker or woman maker, you need two kettlebells of the same size (the kettlebells need to be at least 26 pounds to support your weight). Make sure you follow the guidelines to mastering each exercise individually before attempting the combination. This exercise takes quite a bit of skill to do correctly, so take the time to master the individual exercises first.

See Chapter 13 for explicit instructions on how to perform the man or woman maker as one smoothly flowing combination. Here's a quick refresher:

1. **Stand with your feet shoulder width apart, and position the kettlebells between your feet; the handles are facing sideways.**

2. **As you push your hips back and reach down to put one hand on each kettlebell, perform a burpee to jump back and down into the renegade-row position and do a push-up (see Figure 16-5a).**

3. **After you do one push-up, perform a renegade row on each side.**

4. **From the renegade-row position, jump forward and up so that the kettle-bells are between your feet and slightly behind you (see Figure 16-5b); keep your hands on the kettlebells as you jump.**

5. **Double clean the kettlebells (see Figure 16-5c).**

6. **Keeping the kettlebells racked, perform a rock-bottom squat by sitting back into your hips, letting your knees bend, keeping your spine neutral, and pulling yourself to the ground.**

7. **As you come up from the squat, press the kettlebells up overhead (see Figure 16-5d).**

8. **Re-rack the kettlebells (refer to Figure 16-5c), bring them back down to the ground between your feet, and, without taking your hands off the handles, repeat the exercise, beginning with Step 2.**

Perform five repetitions of the man or woman maker.

Programs for back-to-back training days

As a weekend warrior, you need to be extra careful not to overdo it with your kettlebell routine. Use the programs in Tables 16-1 and 16-2 as a guideline when you're training on back-to-back days. In terms of length, your workouts can be anywhere from 30 to 45 minutes each. Be sure to keep your repetition count low for the intense combinations — anywhere from five to ten repetitions is plenty with a set count of three to four and a 30- to

45-second rest break in between exercises. Alternate between the two training options in the tables to make sure your program is balanced and stays challenging.

Don't forget to warm up and cool down! Choose two or three of the stretches and one of the kettlebell exercises I describe in Chapter 5 for your warm-up. Also, be sure to do at least one of the cool-down exercises I describe in that chapter after your main workout.

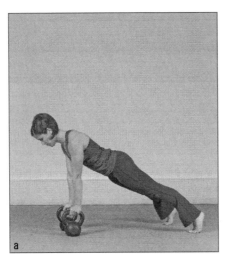

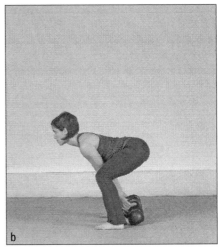

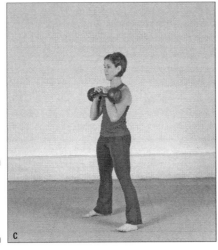

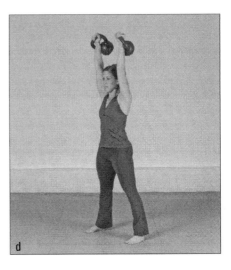

Figure 16-5:
The man
or woman
maker.

Table 16-1	Weekend-Warrior Training Option 1				
Saturday			**Sunday**		
Exercise	**Number of Reps and Sets**	**Reference Chapter**	**Exercise**	**Number of Reps and Sets**	**Reference Chapter**
Two-arm swing	10, 4	6	Single-leg dead lift/ one-arm row combo	8, 4	10, 13
Clean/squat/ press combo	10, 4	8, 9	Body weight squats	20, 4	5
Renegade row with two kettlebells	10, 4	11	Two-arm swing	10, 4	6

Table 16-2	Weekend-Warrior Training Option 2				
Saturday			**Sunday**		
Exercise	**Number of Reps and Sets**	**Reference Chapter**	**Exercise**	**Number of Reps and Sets**	**Reference Chapter**
Man or woman maker	5, 3	5, 8, 11, 13	Single-leg dead lift/ one-arm row combo	10, 4	10, 13
Two-arm swing	10, 3	6	Push-up to *T*-Hold	5, 4	5
			Two-arm swing	10, 4	6

Chapter 17

Rehabbing or Supporting Substantial Weight Loss with Kettlebells

. . . .

In This Chapter
▶ Using kettlebells to recover from an injury
▶ Losing lots of weight with the help of kettlebells

. . . .

An essential final step in recovering from any injury is strength training the affected area of your body. The kettlebell exercises in the first part of this chapter are great examples of exercises that strengthen multiple muscle groups at once; you can use them as part of your rehabilitation during the strength-training phase of your recovery.

Kettlebells are also useful when you have a substantial amount of weight to lose (or when you've already started losing a lot of weight); in fact, kettlebells are probably one of the most effective training tools at your disposal. Take a look at the second part of this chapter for some exercises you can use to fight the fat.

Using Kettlebells As You Recover from an Injury

Basic kettlebell exercises, done properly, are a powerful tool to use during the remodeling phase of your injury recovery because the movements mimic your everyday-life movements. So not only do you re-strengthen the area of injury, but you also move about your everyday life with a lot more strength and confidence. The exercises in this section, which address common areas of injury, like the shoulder, knee, and back, focus on using light kettlebells to get back your strength, mobility, and flexibility. Just be sure to consult your doctor about using kettlebells before you begin a workout routine.

The exercises in this section are for those of you who have already gone through physical therapy and have your doctor's clearance to strength train. They aren't appropriate for those of you who have just sustained an injury and haven't yet gone through physical therapy; going through a doctor's prescribed physical therapy plan is the first step in getting healthy again. Physical therapy helps ease you back into the appropriate exercises and ranges of motion for your specific injury — only after doing so can you safely start a kettlebell routine.

If you've gone through a major surgery, make sure to talk to your doctor and physical therapist about designing a strength-training program for you. The exercises illustrated in this section are most appropriate for people who have sustained minor and common injuries, not people who have had major surgery.

Getting your doctor's clearance and finding a trainer

Work closely with your physical therapist or doctor to determine whether kettlebell exercises are appropriate for recovering from your particular injury. Chances are that if your injury is of a typical variety, your practitioner will want you to engage in a modified strength-training routine, and kettlebells will do the trick. Be sure to explain to your doctor exactly what kettlebells are and how they're different from traditional strength-training programs (refer to Chapter 2 for an explanation of the differences). Follow your doctor's advice because he or she knows your medical history best.

In addition to consulting with your doctor and physical therapist, you should seek the expertise of an RKC-certified instructor who has experience working with an injury like yours. See the appendix for more on finding an RKC.

Trying three all-around rehab exercises

The two-arm swing, half or full Turkish get-up, and single-leg dead lift are good all-around rehab exercises because they work most of your major muscle groups and ranges of motion. If you have an upper- or lower-body injury, these three exercises can help you feel strong and mobile again without overstressing the injured area.

While you exercise, make sure you listen to your body. If something doesn't feel right, stop the exercise immediately and consult with your practitioner.

The modified two-arm swing

If you suffer from nonspecific low-back pain, have knee or ankle problems, or have an upper-body injury, you can do a modified version of the two-arm swing to get your body moving and feeling strong again. The form and movements for this version of the two-arm swing are the same as those for the traditional two-arm swing (see Chapter 6); you simply modify this exercise by using a lighter kettlebell that's about 14 to 18 pounds. Just make sure you master the hip, spine, and breathing techniques in Chapters 4 and 5 before moving on to the two-arm swing.

Chapter 6 explains all the details for how to properly execute the two-arm swing; I provide the basics here: Stand with your feet shoulder width apart, and reach down to put two hands on the kettlebell. Swing the kettlebell behind you (like you're hiking a football; see Figure 17-1a), and aggressively snap your hips forward as you stand up tall. Drive through your heels, extend your spine, and squeeze your thighs, glutes, and abs as you bring your arms and kettlebell to stomach or chest height (see Figure 17-1b).

Perform ten repetitions.

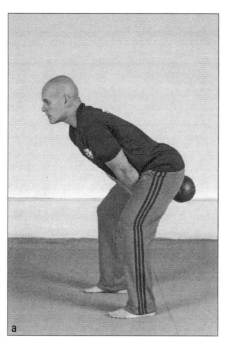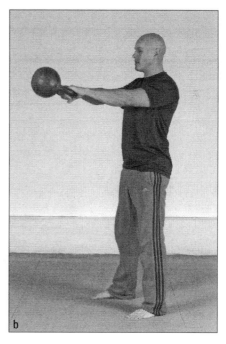

Figure 17-1:
The two-arm swing.

a

b

The half Turkish get-up

Depending on your injury, the half or full Turkish get-up (TGU) can be a powerful exercise for increasing shoulder mobility and flexibility. Begin with a very light kettlebell; a 10-pound bell is a good starting point.

Be sure to start with the half TGU before moving on to the full version (I describe both versions in detail in Chapter 7). Here are the basics for the half version: Lie on your back, holding the kettlebell with both hands at your chest. Bend your left knee to a 90-degree angle, press the kettlebell up, locking out your left elbow, and release your right hand. Using your right elbow and hand to help you, aggressively sit up at a 45-degree angle (see Figure 17-2a). Come to a fully upright, seated position (see Figure 17-2b). Then, slowly and in a controlled motion, lie back down to the start position.

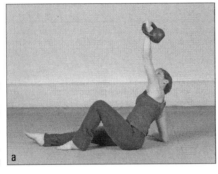 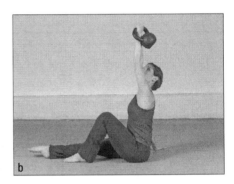

Figure 17-2:
The half
Turkish
get-up.

Perform two repetitions on your left side; then set down the kettlebell and pass it behind your body or move your body around the kettlebell to switch sides. Perform two repetitions on the right side.

If you have a knee injury, the full Turkish get-up may not be appropriate for you because you have to put your weight on one knee during the lunge phase of the full Turkish get-up. In that case, practice only the half Turkish get-up.

The single-leg dead lift

Perhaps one of the best exercises for recovering from a knee or ankle injury is the single-leg dead lift. This exercise works to strengthen the joints and tendons around the affected area while limiting your ability to overcompensate with other parts of the body.

Chapter 10 provides all the details on how to perform the single-leg dead lift; however, when you're using the single-leg dead lift for rehabilitation, start by doing a nonweighted, chair-supported version. To do this modified version, stand with your feet slightly apart, place one hand on a chair back, and lift your left leg off the ground and behind you. Slowly sit back into your hips and descend as far as your current flexibility allows you to go (see Figure 17-3). In a controlled movement, drive through your right heel as you exhale, and stand up tall, pinching your abs and glutes as you do so.

After you master the basic movements, progress to the weighted version of the single-leg dead lift with a light kettlebell (the size you use for the two-arm swing — 14 to 18 pounds — works well). See Chapter 10 for instructions.

Perform five repetitions on your left side; then switch sides and perform five repetitions on your right side.

Taking it easy and avoiding certain exercises

Although you may feel really good as you move through the preceding exercises, your body will get the most benefit during the first part of your strength-training rehab phase if you don't try to overdo it. In other words, don't use heavy weights or attempt to do exercises that aren't appropriate for this phase of your healing. A good rule of thumb is to begin with a light weight and do two to three sets of each exercise. You can then progress to 50 to 75 percent of the intensity you used in your pre-injury workout routines.

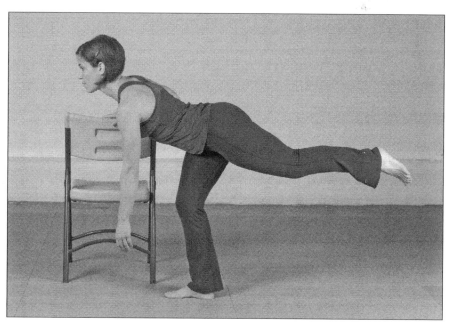

Figure 17-3:
The single-leg dead lift.

Use the sample workout routine in Table 17-1 as a guideline during your strength-training rehab phase, along with the exercises your physical therapist gives you. Use the Z-Health warm-up options I offer in Chapter 5 to get your body ready for your workout. In addition, if your specific injury allows you to move through the ranges of motion for the dynamic warm-up options from that chapter, choose two of them to further prepare your body for exercise.

Table 17-1	A Sample Rehab Routine			
Exercise	Number of Reps in Each Set	Rest Period between Sets	Number of Sets	Reference Chapter
Half Turkish get-up on the left	2 to 3	30 seconds	1 to 2	7
Half Turkish get-up on the right	2 to 3	30 seconds	1 to 2	7
Two-arm swing	10	30 seconds	2 to 3	6
Single-leg dead lift on the left	5 to 8	20 seconds	2 to 3	10
Single-leg dead lift on the right	5 to 8	20 seconds	2 to 3	10

As you grow stronger, you can add a one-arm row, which I describe in Chapter 10, to the routine in Table 17-1; you can use the same size weight you use for swings for this exercise.

Don't forget to cool down properly after you finish your workout routine. Choose a few of the Z-Health options I provide in Chapter 5, or do any of the cool-down stretches I describe in that chapter that your specific injury allows you to move through without pain.

For the beginning phase of your strength-training rehab routine, stay away from exercises that explore ranges of motion that aren't appropriate for your specific injury, like deep squats, heavy military presses, or snatches. In addition, don't use weight that's too heavy; if you can't perform five to eight reps of an exercise without struggling or straining, the weight is too heavy. Talk to your doctor if you're unsure of whether an exercise is appropriate for you or if you're trying to decide on the proper size kettlebell to use.

Supporting Major Weight Loss with Kettlebells

If you have a substantial amount of weight to lose (or if you're in the process of losing a lot of weight) and you've tried different exercise routines with little success, kettlebells may be just the workout you need to boost your metabolism and fight the fat. Over the years, I've worked with a handful of individuals who wanted to lose 100 pounds or more, and I can tell you that you can use kettlebells to help you lose weight — even if you've never lifted a weight before. Like the individuals I've worked with, I bet you'll find working out with kettlebells to be fun and challenging. Best of all, you don't have to spend two hours a day in the gym working out to see a difference. All you need is the willingness to learn a new routine and the discipline to consistently follow your new kettlebell program. Although the discipline part is hard for everyone, many people who use kettlebells find them addicting.

Kettlebells are an effective tool for major weight loss because

- ✔ Kettlebell exercises are easy on the joints and tendons — no running or jumping involved!

- ✔ Kettlebells have been proven to burn lots of calories in short periods of time.

- ✔ Kettlebell exercises are made up of natural movements and are easy to learn.

- ✔ Kettlebell exercises are easy to do in the privacy of your home — which is a big bonus if you're self-conscious about going to the gym.

- ✔ Mastering the exercises requires no previous weight-lifting experience or athletic fitness level.

Part of being successful in losing weight and keeping it off is strength training to build muscle and get rid of fat, which is what you do with your kettlebell workout. Compared to traditional weights, kettlebells offer you the bonus of having to spend less time working out to see the same — or better — results. So give your new kettlebell workout a try using the modifications I describe in this section (with your doctor's permission, of course). You'll begin to see and feel results very quickly, which will encourage you to continue. And, who knows, you just might become addicted, too!

Getting your doctor's clearance

You absolutely must speak with your doctor about the kettlebell workout you want to perform before beginning the program. Most likely, your doctor has recommended that you exercise and strength train, but it's always important for you to meet with your doctor before beginning any new workout program. Your doctor knows your medical history and can help you decide whether the kettlebell workout is a good fit for you. In addition, ask your doctor to specify how often you should strength train and how long each workout should last.

Sizzling the fat with three great exercises

Use the exercise modifications in this section to guide you as you start your kettlebell workout routine. In addition, use the sample workout routine in the later section "Putting together a safe program" to begin to consistently do your kettlebell workout throughout the week. Begin the exercises in this section with a light kettlebell between 10 and 14 pounds for women and between 14 and 18 pounds for men.

The towel swing

If you're looking to shed the pounds but can't quite get the kettlebell between your legs and back up again during the two-arm swing (an exercise I describe in Chapter 6), you can use the *towel swing* to help you swing the kettlebell between your legs and hinge back properly with your hips. The towel in this exercise acts as a handle lengthener.

The towel swing isn't any less effective than the two-arm swing (without a towel), so this modification gives you all the same benefits of the unmodified exercise while keeping your form in check.

Before you begin, turn to Chapters 4 and 5 for the proper hip, spine, and breathing techniques, and then move on to Chapter 6 for all the details on performing the towel swing, which is often used as a corrective exercise for people who aren't sitting back into their hips the right way.

Here are the basics: Stand with your feet shoulder width apart and the kettlebell on the ground between your feet; place the towel through the kettlebell's handle so you have two "handles." Pin your elbows into your rib cage, swing the kettlebell behind you (see Figure 17-4a), and aggressively snap your hips forward as you stand up tall. Drive through your heels, extend your spine, and squeeze your thighs, glutes, and abs as you bring your arms and kettlebell to midstomach height (see Figure 17-4b).

Perform five repetitions.

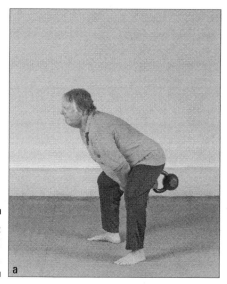 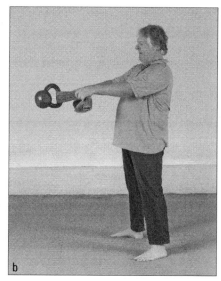

a   b

Figure 17-4:
The towel
swing.

The half Turkish get-up

The half Turkish get-up (TGU) offers many benefits to someone who's looking to shed the pounds. It helps you gain shoulder strength, flexibility, and mobility and works your core muscles — just to name a few.

Chapter 7 has the whole scoop on doing the half TGU, but I provide the basics here: Lie on your back, holding the kettlebell with both hands at your chest. Bend your left knee to a 90-degree angle, press the kettlebell up, locking out your left elbow, and release your right hand (see Figure 17-5a). Using your right elbow and hand to help you, aggressively sit up at a 45-degree angle (see Figure 17-5b). Come to a fully upright, seated position. Then, slowly and in a controlled motion, lie back down to the start position.

As you gain confidence in doing the half TGU, you can progress toward the full TGU, which I describe in detail in Chapter 7, by gradually adding in the steps of that exercise.

Perform two repetitions on your left side; then set down the kettlebell and pass it behind your body or move your body around the kettlebell to switch sides. Perform two repetitions on the right side.

The box squat

When it comes to working your legs, your goal is to be able to squat past 90 degrees in the front squat (see Chapter 8). But if you're carrying a significant amount of extra weight, try practicing the box squat instead. It offers many of the same benefits as the front squat, like working your glutes, thighs, and abs, but also ensures that you don't descend too far and hurt yourself.

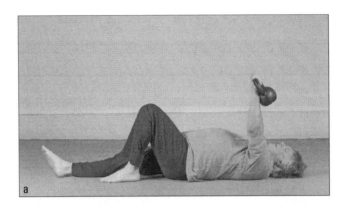

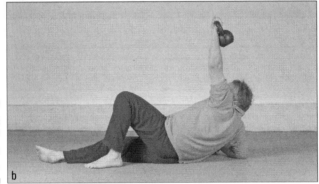

Figure 17-5:
The half
Turkish
get-up.

As the name implies, you need a small, sturdy box to do this exercise (a 16-
to 24-inch box works well for people trying to lose a lot of weight). Flip to
Chapter 8 for details on doing the box squat; I provide the basics here: Place
your box behind you and take a half or full step forward. Stand with your feet
slightly wider than shoulder width apart, your toes pointed slightly out, and
your arms holding your kettlebell by the horns at chest height. With your
weight on your heels, sit back into your hips, letting your knees bend as you
slowly pull yourself to the box (see Figure 17-6). With your weight pushing
through your heels and your knees and core stable, drive up to a fully standing position, with your spine tall and glutes pinched.

If the box you have is too low for you, you can pile up towels to make the seat
higher. Remember, during your squat, you want to only tap your butt to the
box and use it as a guide. As you become stronger and more flexible, you can
remove one towel per workout until you can reach your box without any
towels. Then, after the box becomes easy to reach, remove it and perform the
front squat that I describe in Chapter 8. Go as low as you comfortably can with
perfect form and no pain or pressure in the knees or back.

Perform five repetitions.

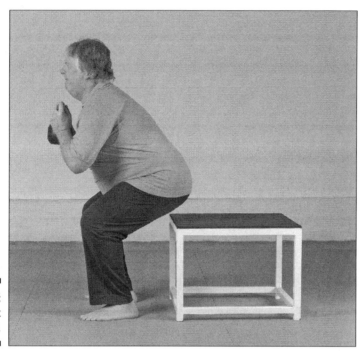

Figure 17-6:
The box
squat.

Putting together a safe program

Begin your kettlebell program slowly with light weights and short 10- to 20-minute workouts, two to three days a week. After you build up your cardiovascular and muscular endurance, you can increase the size kettlebell you use (see Chapter 3) and increase your workout time up to 30 to 45 minutes, three to five days a week. Sounds doable, right? Well, it is!

Use the sample routine in Table 17-2 as a guideline as you begin to work out with kettlebells. Before you start this routine (or any other), be sure to warm up with the three dynamic stretches in Chapter 5, taking care to prepare your body for exercise. After you're comfortable doing the dynamic warm-up stretches, take some time to try one of the warm-up options with the kettlebell, like the halo, or one of the Z-Health options, like knee circles (these warm-up exercises and more are in Chapter 5). Decide which warm-up combination works best for you, and use it before each of your workouts. Keep in mind that the idea is not to wear yourself out before you begin your workout, so don't spend more than five to eight minutes warming up.

Table 17-2	A Sample Routine to Support Major Weight Loss			
Exercise	**Number of Reps in Each Set**	**Rest Period between Sets**	**Number of Sets**	**Reference Chapter**
Half Turkish get–up on the left	2	30 seconds	1 to 2	7
Half Turkish get–up on the right	2	30 seconds	1 to 2	7
Towel swing	5	20 to 30 seconds	2 to 3	6
Box squat	5	30 to 45 seconds	2 to 3	8

Be sure to cool down after your workout with any of the cool-down options I describe in Chapter 5.

After the program in Table 17-2 becomes less challenging for you, try adding in the one-arm row from Chapter 10 and the clean and press exercises from Chapter 8. Additionally, you can increase the number of reps and sets you do and the size kettlebell you use while decreasing the rest period between exercises for even more of a challenge. After you're confident with this program, refer to the workouts in Chapters 9 and 13 to rev up your workouts and take your fitness and health to the next level.

Until you've worked up to a level of conditioning at which you can work out for as long as 20 to 30 minutes with kettlebells and not feel like you're going to fall over or pass out, stay away from the following exercises. If you try to do them before you take off some excess weight, you risk overstressing your joints, which can lead to injury and setbacks in your weight-loss program.

✔ High swings

✔ Full Turkish get-ups

✔ Deep squats

Also avoid adding high-impact exercises (like running and jumping) to your routine until you can do so without risking injury and pain. To determine whether it's safe to add these exercises, ask your doctor. Your kettlebell routine, along with lower-impact exercise programs like walking, yoga, or Pilates, will give you plenty of caloric burn to lose weight safely.

Part V
The Part of Tens

The 5th Wave   By Rich Tennant

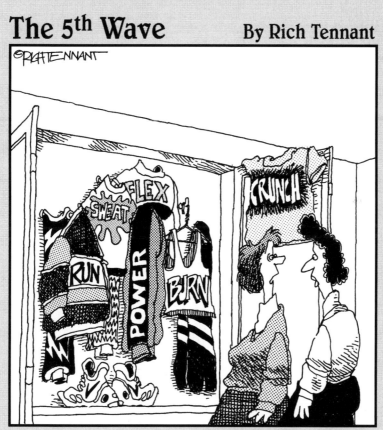

"I'm not sure I can live up to my workout clothes."

In this part . . .

This fun little part offers you tidbits of information that you may be curious about, including ten ways to set and achieve your fitness goals and (nearly) ten tips for working with a certified kettlebell trainer. In addition, I include an appendix, which is packed full of kettlebell resources that can help you increase your knowledge of kettlebells and find a qualified trainer near you.

Chapter 18

Ten Ways to Set and Meet Your Kettlebell Fitness Goals

*O*ver the years, I've watched a handful of students start a kettlebell program with a lot of enthusiasm and good intentions only to fizzle out and quit the program within a few months. As a trainer and business owner, I used to take it quite personally when my students quit. I soon realized, though, that no matter how good the kettlebell routine or program was, if the students didn't have measurable, concrete goals to begin with, they had a hard time sticking with it. The same goes for you — if you don't have a map to guide you, chances are you'll get lost along the way and turn back to what's familiar (that is, whatever exercise or lack of exercise you did in the past).

Goals are important when it comes to any fitness plan because, without them, you don't know where you're going (the end result) or how to get there (the frequency, duration, and other similar characteristics of your workouts). And you certainly don't know how to stay motivated when things don't work out perfectly as planned (which is almost never).

So how do you set and meet your kettlebell fitness goals? Doing so is actually quite simple and takes only a small amount of preparation time on your part. In this chapter, I outline ten ways to set and meet your goals; my suggestions here fall into the following three categories:

▶ **Mental preparation:** Mental preparation is an important part of setting your kettlebell fitness goals, and taking some time to go through this process before you start your kettlebell routine is key in helping you reach what you set out to accomplish. I remember when I wanted to change my body fat percentage and get myself into the best shape possible. I started by going through the mental preparation processes that I describe in the first three sections of this chapter. After I prepared my mind for the task at hand, everything else flowed quite easily.

✓ **Research preparation:** Your research preparation includes any items you need to get more information on before you begin your program. Your preworkout research is another important part of your overall road map because it solidifies the mental prep you previously did and keeps you moving forward toward your goal. The most time-consuming research task I suggest in this chapter is planning your meals, but the other two prep items (having your body fat tested and finding a trainer) don't take long at all.

✓ **Workout action:** The last four sections in this chapter describe the four actions you need to take to execute your fitness plan. At this point, you'll have done all the mental and research preparation you needed to do in order to begin, so it's time to get started!

Be Specific about Your Goals

What do you want to accomplish with your new kettlebell fitness routine? Defining what your measurable goals are is the first crucial step toward accomplishing them. Typically, when I ask clients what their goals are, they tell me they want to lose weight. Sometimes they specify how much weight (the last 10 pounds, for example); other times, they tell me they want to "get in shape" for a special event that's coming up. But, beyond these broad ideas, they don't have a specific plan to reach their goals — other than to begin a workout program.

Here are some common goals to help you think about your own specific goals:

✓ Lose body fat.

✓ Gain strength and power.

✓ Increase lean muscle mass.

✓ Increase cardiovascular and muscle endurance.

✓ Feel better and less stressed.

Which of these goals do you want to reach? After you decide on your overall goal, grab a notebook and pen and write it down (use this notebook only for your kettlebell fitness goals and label it as such). If what you want to accomplish isn't on this list, take some time to think about your specific goal, and write it in your notebook before you start your routine.

Find a workout partner. Perhaps a friend wants to start a new fitness routine or has a fitness goal similar to yours. Reach out to your friend and ask him or her to start a kettlebell fitness program with you. But remember, if your partner doesn't show up often or doesn't motivate you in some way, just work out on your own or find a new partner.

Write Out Your Kettlebell Road Map

After you write down what you want to accomplish through your fitness program, you need to design a road map for how to get there. To complete your road map, answer the following five questions (jot down your answers now):

- ✔ What days will you work out?
- ✔ What time of day will you work out?
- ✔ Where will you work out?
- ✔ How many days per week will you work out and for how long?
- ✔ What size kettlebell will you need?

There's no point in setting unrealistic goals. Know yourself and your habits, and use that info as a starting point. If you're someone who hits the snooze button a few (or many) times before getting out of bed, don't choose to work out before your day starts (if you do, chances are good that you'll snooze right past your workout on more than one occasion). On the other hand, if you often get sidetracked on your way home from work or typically like to get home quickly after leaving the office, perhaps working out before you go to work is the best option for you. Decide what's best for you, and write out your road map.

Set Up Your Workout Area

After you decide where you're going to work out as part of your kettlebell road map, gather your equipment and anything else you need to be successful with your program. I suggest beginning this process a week ahead of your scheduled start date so you don't have to rush; if you decide to start your new kettlebell fitness routine on Monday morning, don't wait until Sunday night to get your equipment, clothing, and area ready. By setting up your workout area ahead of time, you get your mind thinking about starting and progressing through your workout routine. In addition, the visual reminder keeps you motivated and excited to follow through with your program. Here are a few suggestions for setting up your workout area if you plan to work out at home (see Chapters 2 and 3 for more details on these topics):

✔ Clean out and organize your workout area, even if it's only a small corner of your office or living room. Remove any clutter.

✔ Buy the right size kettlebell for you and a stopwatch.

✔ Purchase the educational material (DVDS or books, for example) that you plan to use for your workouts (definitely keep this one handy!).

✔ Buy a blank notebook, label it as your workout log, and make sure to keep a pen or pencil with it in your workout area.

Your workout log is a very important part of your routine; try to record every workout you do in your notebook. Include the exercises you did, the repetitions and sets you performed, and the size of kettlebell you used.

✔ Prepare your floor surface by purchasing and laying down a large yoga mat or martial arts floor tiles.

✔ Make sure you have comfortable workout clothes that fit you well.

✔ Make your area inspiring and appealing by putting up a photo or quote that helps motivate and inspire you, having music nearby, and having a basket filled with workout towels and bottled water.

If you plan to take your kettlebell to a gym or outside, prepare your gym bag to include your kettlebell, workout log, stopwatch, water, towel, workout clothes, and anything else you may need.

Have Your Body Fat Tested

Although getting your body fat tested can be a bit intimidating, it's an essential part of your workout preparation because your body fat percentage is the best measurable starting point you have.

Because you can't get your body fat percentage from your home scale, you need to find a certified body fat tester (typically an independent company). Find a tester who uses the *hydrostatic* (under water) method or body fat calipers; they're the most affordable and accurate methods available today (although each method has a small margin of error). Both tests should be done in a private area with just you, the tester, and anyone who needs to be there to support you.

I recommend taking the plunge and getting dunked with the hydrostatic method because this method gives you detailed information on what your body fat percentage and weight are, what the normal range is, and how much fat you need to lose to be in your desired range. Body fat calipers are a good alternative if the hydrostatic method isn't available in your area, but they aren't as accurate and will provide you with only a body fat percentage range.

Write down your current body fat percentage and weight under the goals section in your kettlebell road map notebook, and, next to them, write your target body fat percentage and weight. After you practice your kettlebell program for at least two to three months, you can get retested to measure your progress.

Plan Your Meals

I don't expect you to spend all weekend cooking for the week ahead, but planning your meals really does help you reach your fitness goals. If you keep a varied but simple diet, planning meals is easy to do.

Everyone has different nutritional needs and considerations, so it's important that you know yours before you start planning your meals. Talk to your doctor, see a nutritionist, or follow the simple tips I offer in this section to find out what your nutritional needs are.

If you have it in your budget, I suggest hiring a nutritionist to help guide you through your first month or two of starting a new kettlebell fitness routine. Make sure the person you hire is at least a clinical nutritionist. Don't rely on personal trainers who don't have any nutritionist credentials to give you specific advice on what to eat and how much to eat. It's well worth the investment to hire a professional, especially if your diet is all out of whack.

If your budget doesn't allow you to hire a nutritionist, you can still plan your meals affordably. Just follow these tips to help you get started:

- ✔ **Create a food journal by sectioning off an area in either your goal notebook or your workout log.** In your food journal, record the nutritional details for each meal, including the number of calories and carbohydrates and the amount of protein and fat. Numerous food dictionaries, such as *The Calorie Counter For Dummies* by Rosanne Rust and Meri Raffetto (Wiley), are available to help you figure out the nutritional intake for almost any food, and many online calorie counters exist, as well. If you use an online version, print out your records and post them in your notebook.

✔ **Invest in a food scale.** Knowing portion size is an important part of planning healthy meals. A food scale is the easiest way to accurately measure portion size.

✔ **Set aside a few minutes at the beginning of the week to decide what you're going to eat that week, and write out your grocery store list accordingly.** You don't need to come up with an elaborate weekly menu; simple is best when it comes to planning your meals. If you need to prepare meals to take with you to work, be sure to include them in your weekly menu and prepare them the night before. Sounds easy right? Well, it is!

Although planning your meals takes some time, keep in mind that you can't outwork a bad diet. If you aren't willing to commit some time to educating yourself on what you should be eating, planning your meals, and writing down what you eat, chances are your workout routine's results won't be nearly as good as they'd be if you took the time to do so.

Find a Certified Instructor

Whether you plan to work out at home, outside, or at your gym, finding a Russian Kettlebell Challenge–certified instructor (RKC) is the best way to begin your kettlebell fitness program. By the time you buy your equipment and anything else you need to get started, you may not have a lot of room in your budget, but, if you can afford it, spend some extra money for training sessions with a good RKC — the benefits will far outweigh the costs. It takes a thousand or more good repetitions to correct one bad one, so, if at all possible, hire an RKC for at least one session to get you started on the right foot.

Look at the full listing of RKCs on the Web site www.dragondoor.com/rkc, and make sure to look at Chapter 19 to get more information on how to find the right RKC for you and how to work well with him or her during your training program. I also provide some resources on trainers in the appendix.

Get Moving!

Armed with your overall goal, your kettlebell road map, and your workout log, you're ready to start your first workout. Throughout this book, I give you many different workout routines to choose from. I suggest that you begin with the beginner workouts and routines I outline in Chapter 9. There's no time like the present, so pick the day and time you want to start and get moving!

Surf the Web for Even More Info

The Internet offers numerous kettlebell-related resources and online communities that help you stay motivated, ask training-related questions, and find like-minded individuals. Here are just some of the things you can do online:

✔ **Get training advice.** The best online community is the Dragon Door forum at www.dragondoor.com, where qualified RKCs are always on hand to give training advice. Here, you can read about different RKCs' training-related experiences and post videos of your form and technique for review.

✔ **Improve your kettlebell routine.** The Internet is home to several excellent blogs written by highly experienced RKCs. These blogs offer tips on form, workouts, and much more and can help you improve the intensity and/or effectiveness of your own kettlebell routine. Here are some of my favorites (check out more in the appendix):

- www.ironcorekettlebells.com

- www.appliedstrength.com

- www.chasingstrength.com

✔ **Find free workouts.** Although you don't need to spend a lot of time online (compared to how much you spend working out), the Internet can be a great place to find good, free workouts and training advice — as long as it's from the right source. YouTube isn't always the best place to find quality training videos, so stick with one of the following resources to make sure you're getting the best advice (you can find more resources in the appendix):

- www.ironcorekettlebells.com

- www.dragondoor.com

- www.appliedstrength.com

Measure Your Progress

One of the reasons why you should record each workout in a log (as I suggest in the earlier section "Set Up Your Workout Area") is to give yourself a record of where you started and how much progress you've made. Typically, students who don't create a workout log don't know how much stronger they've become unless I point it out to them. Keeping a workout log allows you to measure how close you've come to reaching your overall goal.

After you've been doing your program consistently for four to six weeks, look back to the first day of your workout log to see where you started; then flip through it to see how far you've come. Maybe you've increased the size of your kettlebell or have been able to work out for longer periods of time; maybe you've added more days to your workout. Or perhaps you aren't making much progress at all. Looking at your workout log, you can assess how you're progressing (or not progressing) and determine where to go next.

In addition, after you've been consistently working out for 8 to 12 weeks, get your body fat tested again using the same method you did for your initial test (see the section "Have Your Body Fat Tested"). Getting your body fat rechecked either reinforces that you're doing everything right or clues you in to where you may need to make changes. If your body fat hasn't changed much since you began your kettlebell program, you need to take a closer look at your diet and your workout log to assess what you're eating and how much you're really working out. Take the time to measure your progress and make any changes you think are necessary.

Keep Your Workouts Fresh

After you've been doing your kettlebell fitness routine for four to six weeks, consider changing some elements of your routine to keep it fresh and help motivate you to continue making progress. To continue to progress with your kettlebell fitness program, do the following:

- **Change your workout routine.** After you've been doing the same routine for a while, take some time to create a new four- to six-week kettlebell road map. Refer to Chapter 13 for some new and challenging workout routines.

- **Use a heavier weight.** Is your kettlebell getting too easy to swing? If so, consider buying a heavier bell. Flip to Chapter 3 for information on picking the right bell for you.

- **Master new exercises.** Although you can never practice the kettlebell basics too much, take some time to learn one or two new exercises, and add them to your routine to keep it fresh.

- **Consider hiring an RKC.** If you didn't hire a trainer to begin with, now may be the right time to do so. Refer to Chapter 19 for tips on finding and working with an RKC.

Chapter 19

Nearly Ten Guidelines for Finding and Working Out with a Certified Trainer

In This Chapter

▶ Finding a qualified kettlebell trainer

▶ Working well with the trainer you choose

*W*orking with a Russian Kettlebell Challenge (RKC)–certified trainer two to three days a week or more, either individually or in a group setting, is a big commitment — financially and mentally — on the part of both you and your trainer. In addition, the person you hire to be your trainer is basically in charge of your body for the duration of your training — making sure it moves properly and reaches its optimal potential (and making sure you don't get hurt!). Keeping you safe and making your workouts as effective as they can be is a huge responsibility and one that you want your trainer to take seriously.

So what should you look for when selecting and working out with your trainer? And how can you be sure you've found the right person for the job? The tips in this chapter are here to help you through the process of choosing and then working out with your trainer.

You pay for every training session you attend, and you need to get out of it what you expect. If a trainer doesn't meet your expectations at any time, speak with him personally. If he doesn't respond to your concerns, move on to find someone who does.

Check the Trainer's Credentials and Experience

What kinds of credentials are important for a kettlebell instructor to have? Most importantly, you want your potential trainer to be an RKC-certified instructor. The RKC has been in existence since 2001 and is the only recognizable kettlebell trainer certification in the United States. The RKC is considered the gold standard in the industry, and you shouldn't trust your body to anyone else. Hiring an RKC trainer ensures that you'll be working with someone who has done all the following:

✔ Passed a rigorous three-day physical challenge during which he demonstrated precise and safe form and technique for foundational kettlebell exercises

✔ Demonstrated good judgment in his own technique and form, especially in terms of safety

✔ Demonstrated good judgment along with precise and effective teaching skills with new students

✔ Passed a grueling snatch test to prove physical readiness and conditioning (see Chapter 12 for details about the snatch exercise)

✔ Passed a graduation workout that also tested physical readiness

✔ Agreed to abide by a professional RKC code of conduct

As kettlebells have gained in popularity, spinoffs of the RKC certification have sprung up from trainers and organizations that just don't have the experience and qualifications to offer a comprehensive kettlebell trainer certification like the RKC. So ask your potential kettlebell instructor to provide you with a copy of his RKC certificate, just to be safe — and if he doesn't have one, find one who does.

Besides being RKC certified, the trainer you hire needs to have at least one year of experience teaching students how to use kettlebells either in a class setting, in a one-on-one setting, or both. From my own experience as a trainer and as a gym owner who has hired countless trainers over the years, a good kettlebell trainer needs at least a year to perfect not only his own form and technique but also his ability to translate both basic and complex instructions in an easy-to-understand format.

If your potential trainer can't get you moving properly with a kettlebell within the first five to ten minutes of your first session (excluding any warm-up), move on to find someone who can. Instructing well comes with the experience of working with many students over time, so even if you find a qualified RKC trainer with less than a year's experience, keep looking until you find one with more.

In addition to following the preceding suggestions, ask your potential kettlebell trainer these questions to see if he's the right fit for you:

- ✔ **What is your typical client type?** In other words, find out whether the trainer specializes in working with athletes, overweight people, young adults, seniors, people rehabbing from injury, pregnant women, or just regular folks who want to exercise. Your potential trainer's client list is important because you want your trainer to have experience working with people like you.

- ✔ **Where do you train your clients? At your own studio, out of another gym, or at your home?** The location needs to be convenient for you; otherwise, you'll have a hard time making it to your workouts as time goes on.

- ✔ **How many clients do you currently have?** If your trainer has at least a year's worth of experience teaching, he should have a well-established client base. In general, you want to hire someone who has worked with at least four to five dozen students on a regular basis in that period of time. Any less than that may signal that the trainer's experience level and breadth of experience is low; in that case, you need to find another trainer.

- ✔ **Do you offer personal training, group classes, or both? How many students are typically in a class, and do you do the workout along with the class or use the time to instruct?** Whether you hire a personal trainer or join group classes is really a matter of preference and budget. An experienced instructor should be able to handle 15 students (or more) in a class at a time, but a smaller class size is always ideal so that you get the personal attention of the instructor throughout your workout. I don't recommend taking a class or hiring a trainer who works out along with you because the trainer's full attention needs to be on you and your class, not on himself.

- ✔ **Do you carry liability insurance?** The trainer you hire should absolutely carry liability insurance because doing so is considered a best practice in the industry and protects both of you in case of an incident.

- ✔ **What other personal-training or class-training certifications do you hold?** Although holding credentials other than the RKC isn't necessary, it's worth asking if your potential trainer has other fitness-related certifications. A certification from a well-recognized fitness organization like the National Strength and Conditioning Association or the American Council on Exercise shows that your trainer has acquired some knowledge about anatomy and the way the body performs.

- ✔ **Have you authored any instructional kettlebell DVDs, books, or articles?** Many experienced trainers have produced kettlebell workout DVDs or written books or articles on kettlebell training. Not all the kettlebell products on the market are worth the money, though, so I offer you some tips on choosing good material in the appendix.

Beware of a Trainer Who Doesn't Ask about Your Health History

One of the first questions your trainer should ask you before teaching you how to use kettlebells is "What's your health history?" To help keep you safe, your trainer needs to know about any previous injuries, surgeries, or any medications you're currently taking. Although this information may seem quite personal to you, you need to tell your trainer anything and everything about your body to help her determine what exercises you need to avoid and what exercises you need to modify.

If your trainer doesn't ask you about prior injuries, beware. Kettlebells are a very dynamic training tool, but they aren't a good fit for everyone. The only way for your trainer to know if kettlebell exercise is appropriate for you is to ask you about your health history. If your trainer doesn't ask, move on and find someone who does.

Watch Out for Nutritional Advice from the Trainer

One of my biggest pet peeves is when trainers offer specific nutritional advice when they don't have the qualifications to do so. Offering general nutritional advice, like telling you to eat enough protein and carbs and to drink lots of water is one thing. But prescribing a specific diet for you is something else entirely.

If your trainer tries to prescribe a diet for you and doesn't have the qualifications to do so, you need to take your business somewhere else. If you need nutritional advice, hire a nutritionist to work with you and your trainer to help you reach your goals. Just because your trainer looks good doesn't mean his diet will work for you.

Set Goals and Measure Progress Together

In addition to asking you about your health history, your trainer should ask you about your personal fitness goals during your first session. (If you don't know what your individual goals are, turn to Chapter 18 for help setting them.) All your training sessions need to focus on helping you reach the goals you set during your first session. For example, if you want to lose ten pounds in eight weeks, your trainer needs to design a workout program that helps you accomplish that goal.

In addition to helping you work toward your goals, your trainer needs to help you monitor and measure your progress. A good way for your trainer to help you measure your progress is to give you a workout log in which you can record personal details (like your starting weight), as well as details about your actual workouts, including the exercise, the number of sets and repetitions, the duration of the workout, and the size kettlebell you used. Over time, a workout log is a perfect way for you and your trainer to determine whether you're meeting your goals. (Flip to Chapter 18 for more about tracking progress and setting goals.)

Find Out How the Trainer Teaches Basic Kettlebell Exercises

If you're interested in joining a group class with a trainer, that trainer should require you to take two to three one-hour individual beginner lessons first. At my gym, Iron Core, I've always implemented this requirement because you can't teach a beginner how to properly use kettlebells while you're trying to instruct a group class of more-experienced students. Although these beginner lessons may be an extra investment, you need them to set the proper foundation for your kettlebell routine. Don't attempt to take a class without first learning the five to six basic exercises that I describe in Part II of this book. Most people need two to three one-hour lessons in a beginner setting to master the basics well enough to do well in a class.

If you start your kettlebell practice in a personal-training session, your trainer has more time to focus on you, which means you can learn the five to six basic exercises within one to two one-hour sessions. You simply can't achieve a solid foundation and get off to a good start in less time.

Assess the Kettlebell Size the Trainer Recommends

The kettlebell size that your trainer recommends needs to be the appropriate one for a beginning student. Typically, females begin with a 14- to 18-pound bell, and men begin with a 26- to 35-pound bell. However, your trainer needs to evaluate your individual circumstances before recommending a starting weight. For example, if you're an overweight male who hasn't exercised in a year or more, you need to start with a lighter weight for your first few sessions. On the other hand, starting with a weight that's too light for your personal fitness level doesn't challenge you to move the weight with proper form.

An experienced trainer knows just the right size weight for you to begin with. However, if you start using a certain kettlebell, and you think it's too heavy or too light, be sure to speak up. Your trainer may need to correct your form to help you use the bell properly or increase or decrease your kettlebell size.

Make Sure the Trainer Focuses on Form and Technique, Not on Counting Reps

You don't want to hire a trainer who simply counts repetitions for you. Although counting reps is part of your trainer's job, focusing on your form and technique and instructing you on how to properly do the exercises are much more important. Even if you have good form, your trainer needs to remind you to keep your form solid and give you cues and motivation to get you through your workouts. Simply counting repetitions doesn't do much for you or your form, and it isn't worth the cost of a session or class.

Determine Whether the Trainer Practices What He or She Preaches

Ultimately, you want to hire a trainer who motivates you to look and feel your best. But you also need to make sure your RKC practices what he preaches. Your trainer may not fit a certain body image, but he should use kettlebells on a regular basis. After all, part of being an experienced trainer is continually working on perfecting form, technique, and teaching points; doing so certainly doesn't come without practice. So, when you're looking for a trainer, should you choose the person who looks best in his gym clothes? Not necessarily, but you do want someone who's committed to his own training (often his physique is a reflection of that commitment).

Appendix

Kettlebell Resources

Are you interested in finding out even more about kettlebells? In this appendix, I provide information on where to find the gear you need and point you toward gyms and instructors in the United States, along with a few other kettlebell-related resources.

Sources for Kettlebells, Workout DVDs, and Downloadable Workouts

To buy the official Russian Kettlebell Challenge (RKC) kettlebell, go to www.ironcorekettlebells.com/shop, or purchase directly from the manufacturer at www.dragondoor.com/kettlebells. If you prefer, you can contact these RKC kettlebell distributors instead:

- ✔ www.kettlebellssouthbay.com (California)
- ✔ www.kettlebility.com/content/products (Washington)
- ✔ www.summitkettlebells.com/buy-kettlebells.html (Texas)

For instant downloadable workouts and workout DVDs, go to

- ✔ www.ironcorekettlebells.com/shop
- ✔ www.dragondoor.com/kettlebells
- ✔ www.Amazon.com

When shopping for a kettlebell workout DVD or online video download, make sure to check that the workout's instructor is RKC certified. If you're looking for beginner workouts, check that the DVD contains an instructional component as well as a workout component. (After you become a more advanced kettlebeller, you can purchase DVDs that have only workouts.) Also, look at the testimonials or reviews from other people who have purchased and used the DVD you're considering. Positive comments about the DVD signal that you're getting a quality product. In terms of price, the average kettlebell DVDs cost between $14.99 and $27.99.

Kettlebell Classes and Personal Trainers near You

The following list of Russian Kettlebell Challenge–certified instructors (often called RKCs) isn't exhaustive by any means, but it's a start. In this list, I include some of the RKCs I've either worked with personally or known someone who's worked with them. If you can find an RKC trainer who's teaching classes or offering personal training in your area, take advantage of that resource. After all, working with a qualified instructor will help keep your form in check and help keep you motivated to continue your workouts.

If you don't see classes in your state here, fear not; you can check out a complete listing of RKC instructors by state at www.dragondoor.com/rkc. You can also contact me with any questions; call me at 858-551-2673 or e-mail me at Sarah@IronCoreKettlebells.com.

California

Classic Iron Kettlebells
Carpinteria, CA 93013
Web site www.classicironkettlebells.com

Girya Kettlebell Training
136 Hamilton Avenue
Palo Alto, CA 94301
Phone 650-273-2637
Web site www.giryastrength.com

Iron Core Kettlebell Strength and Conditioning, North County Location
2128 Thibodo Court
Vista, CA 92081
Phone 858-551-2673
Web site www.ironcorekettlebells.com

Iron Core Kettlebell Strength and Conditioning, Pacific Beach Location
2949 Garnet Avenue
San Diego, CA 92109
Phone 858-551-2673
Web site www.ironcorekettlebells.com

Russian River Kettlebells
424 Moore Lane
Healdsburg, CA 95448
Web site www.russianriverkettlebells.com

Georgia

Condition Kettlebell Gym
659 Auburn Avenue, Unit 157
Atlanta, GA 30312
Phone 404-380-1111
Web site www.gymcondition.com

Illinois

Rhodes Fusion Fitness
538 N. Western Avenue
Chicago, IL 60612
Phone 312-637-9772
Web site www.rhodesfusionfitness.com

Minnesota

Kettlebell Fitness
St. Paul and Minneapolis, MN
Web site www.kettlebellfitness.com

Kinetic Edge Performance, Inc.
683 Bielenberg Drive
Woodbury, MN 55125
Phone 651-330-9319
Web site www.kineticedgeperformance.com

New Mexico

Firebellz
6203 Osuna NE
Albuquerque, NM 87109
Web site www.fire-bellz.com

New York

Five Points Academy
277 Canal Street
New York, NY 10013
Phone 212-226-4474
Web site www.academyfivepoints.com

North Carolina

Rapid Results Fitness
4125 Durham-Chapel Hill Boulevard
Durham, NC 27707
Phone 919-403-8651
Web site www.rapidresultsfitness.net

Pennsylvania

Applied Strength
Pittsburgh, PA
Web site www.appliedstrength.com

Tennessee

Tennessee Kettlebell
256 Seaboard Lane, E-102
Franklin, TN 37067
Web site www.tennesseekettlebell.com

Texas

Texas Kettlebell Club
2331 State Hwy. 46 N
Suite 500
Seguin, TX 78155
Phone 830-556-4180
Web site www.texaskettlebellclub.com

Washington

Kettlebility
905 NE Sixty-fifth Street
Seattle, WA 98115
Phone 206-293-0009
Web site www.kettlebility.com

Wisconsin

TNT Performance
17495 W. Capitol Drive
Suite C
Brookfield, WI 53045
Phone 262-873-0656
Web site www.tntperformancetraining.com

Other Resources for Working Out with Kettlebells

Although one kettlebell is all you need for a simple and effective workout, at some point, you may want to mix in other workout training tools to add more variety and challenge to your routine. To help you spice up your routine, I list some of my favorite training tools here, with Web site addresses, so you can find what you need quickly and easily:

- ✔ **BOSU:** If you want to mix up your warm-ups and workout routines or just add more balance and stability training to your workouts, the BOSU is a good tool to add to your home gym. Each BOSU includes an instructional DVD to help you get started. Go to www.bosufitness. com for more info.

- ✔ **Flooring:** If you want to invest in some special workout flooring for your home gym, check out Great Mats at www.greatmats.com. It has workout mats in varying thicknesses and colors to meet your needs.

- ✔ **Free stuff, special offers, and more:** I've created a page on my Web site especially for *For Dummies* readers (www.ironcorekettlebells. com/dummies); it's packed full of resources to help you further your kettlebell journey.

- **Gymboss workout timer:** The Gymboss workout timer is your best investment (aside from your kettlebell) because it's easy to use and compact; you can lay it on the floor in front of you so you can see it easily or clip it to your waist for easy access during your workouts. Check out www.gymboss.com for more info.

- **Medicine balls:** You can mix up your workout routine a lot just by including medicine balls in some of your exercises; squats, the clean and press, and abdominal-specific exercises lend themselves nicely to using medicine balls. Check out *Dr. Donald Chu's Plyometric Exercises with the Medicine Ball,* Second Edition (www.donchu.com), or go to www.d-ball.com to purchase medicine balls.

- **Nutritionist:** If you're interested in finding a qualified nutritionist in your area who can help you meet your fitness goals through food (see Chapter 18), check out www.sportsnutritionsociety.org/nutritionist.aspx, a Web site that makes it easy to find nutritionists by state.

- **Yoga mats, jump ropes, stability balls, stretch bands or straps, foam rollers, and other extra equipment:** If you're looking to add even more variety to your kettlebell routine, consider purchasing some of the additional equipment I mention throughout this book. Amazon.com carries all this equipment and more; as an added bonus, you can read reviews from people who have used and purchased the product to help you pick out what's best for you.

- **Z-Health:** The Z-Health exercise system offers some good exercises for warming up and cooling down for your kettlebell workouts (check out www.zhealth.net for more details; also see Chapter 5).

Index

• *L* •

Business/Accounting & Bookkeeping

Bookkeeping For Dummies
978-0-7645-9848-7

eBay Business
All-in-One For Dummies,
2nd Edition
978-0-470-38536-4

Job Interviews
For Dummies,
3rd Edition
978-0-470-17748-8

Resumes For Dummies,
5th Edition
978-0-470-08037-5

Stock Investing
For Dummies,
3rd Edition
978-0-470-40114-9

Successful Time
Management
For Dummies
978-0-470-29034-7

Computer Hardware

BlackBerry For Dummies,
3rd Edition
978-0-470-45762-7

Computers For Seniors
For Dummies
978-0-470-24055-7

iPhone For Dummies,
2nd Edition
978-0-470-42342-4

Laptops For Dummies,
3rd Edition
978-0-470-27759-1

Macs For Dummies,
10th Edition
978-0-470-27817-8

Cooking & Entertaining

Cooking Basics
For Dummies,
3rd Edition
978-0-7645-7206-7

Wine For Dummies,
4th Edition
978-0-470-04579-4

Diet & Nutrition

Dieting For Dummies,
2nd Edition
978-0-7645-4149-0

Nutrition For Dummies,
4th Edition
978-0-471-79868-2

Weight Training
For Dummies,
3rd Edition
978-0-471-76845-6

Digital Photography

Digital Photography
For Dummies,
6th Edition
978-0-470-25074-7

Photoshop Elements 7
For Dummies
978-0-470-39700-8

Gardening

Gardening Basics
For Dummies
978-0-470-03749-2

Organic Gardening
For Dummies,
2nd Edition
978-0-470-43067-5

Green/Sustainable

Green Building
& Remodeling
For Dummies
978-0-470-17559-0

Green Cleaning
For Dummies
978-0-470-39106-8

Green IT For Dummies
978-0-470-38688-0

Health

Diabetes For Dummies,
3rd Edition
978-0-470-27086-8

Food Allergies
For Dummies
978-0-470-09584-3

Living Gluten-Free
For Dummies
978-0-471-77383-2

Hobbies/General

Chess For Dummies,
2nd Edition
978-0-7645-8404-6

Drawing For Dummies
978-0-7645-5476-6

Knitting For Dummies,
2nd Edition
978-0-470-28747-7

Organizing For Dummies
978-0-7645-5300-4

SuDoku For Dummies
978-0-470-01892-7

Home Improvement

Energy Efficient Homes
For Dummies
978-0-470-37602-7

Home Theater
For Dummies,
3rd Edition
978-0-470-41189-6

Living the Country Lifestyle
All-in-One For Dummies
978-0-470-43061-3

Solar Power Your Home
For Dummies
978-0-470-17569-9

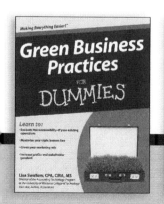

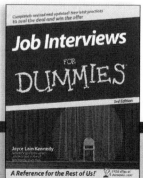

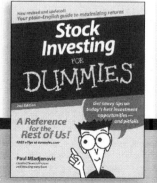

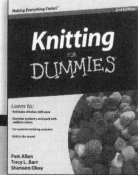

Internet

Blogging For Dummies,
2nd Edition
978-0-470-23017-6

eBay For Dummies,
6th Edition
978-0-470-49741-8

Facebook For Dummies
978-0-470-26273-3

Google Blogger
For Dummies
978-0-470-40742-4

Web Marketing
For Dummies,
2nd Edition
978-0-470-37181-7

WordPress For Dummies,
2nd Edition
978-0-470-40296-2

Language & Foreign Language

French For Dummies
978-0-7645-5193-2

Italian Phrases
For Dummies
978-0-7645-7203-6

Spanish For Dummies
978-0-7645-5194-9

Spanish For Dummies,
Audio Set
978-0-470-09585-0

Macintosh

Mac OS X Snow Leopard
For Dummies
978-0-470-43543-4

Math & Science

Algebra I For Dummies,
2nd Edition
978-0-470-55964-2

Biology For Dummies
978-0-7645-5326-4

Calculus For Dummies
978-0-7645-2498-1

Chemistry For Dummies
978-0-7645-5430-8

Microsoft Office

Excel 2007 For Dummies
978-0-470-03737-9

Office 2007 All-in-One
Desk Reference
For Dummies
978-0-471-78279-7

Music

Guitar For Dummies,
2nd Edition
978-0-7645-9904-0

iPod & iTunes
For Dummies,
6th Edition
978-0-470-39062-7

Piano Exercises
For Dummies
978-0-470-38765-8

Parenting & Education

Parenting For Dummies,
2nd Edition
978-0-7645-5418-6

Type 1 Diabetes
For Dummies
978-0-470-17811-9

Pets

Cats For Dummies,
2nd Edition
978-0-7645-5275-5

Dog Training For Dummies,
2nd Edition
978-0-7645-8418-3

Puppies For Dummies,
2nd Edition
978-0-470-03717-1

Religion & Inspiration

The Bible For Dummies
978-0-7645-5296-0

Catholicism For Dummies
978-0-7645-5391-2

Women in the Bible
For Dummies
978-0-7645-8475-6

Self-Help & Relationship

Anger Management
For Dummies
978-0-470-03715-7

Overcoming Anxiety
For Dummies
978-0-7645-5447-6

Sports

Baseball For Dummies,
3rd Edition
978-0-7645-7537-2

Basketball For Dummies,
2nd Edition
978-0-7645-5248-9

Golf For Dummies,
3rd Edition
978-0-471-76871-5

Web Development

Web Design All-in-One
For Dummies
978-0-470-41796-6

Windows Vista

Windows Vista
For Dummies
978-0-471-75421-3

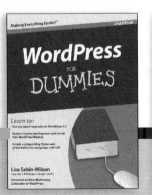
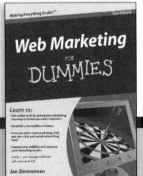
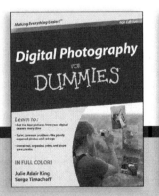
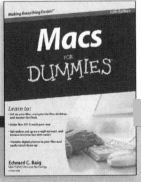

Printed in Great Britain
by Amazon

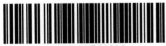

57467532R00206